DIAGNOSED WITH

ALZHEIMER'S

OR

ANOTHER DEMENTIA

KATE SWAFFER & LEE-FAY LOW

About the Authors

A young Kate Swaffer jokingly said to one of her nursing friends, 'Watch out, that'll be us one day, sitting together in the nursing home, not remembering each other!' Ironically, Kate worked as a nurse in a dedicated dementia unit, the first one in South Australia in the 70s; of course she did not realise at that time she would be diagnosed with a younger onset dementia at the age of 49, as a working mum with two teenage children.

Kate Swaffer is a retired nurse, a global advocate and activist for dementia, and is embarking on a PhD in dementia. She co-founded Dementia Alliance International (DAI), the global peak body for people with dementia. As its chair and CEO, and to represent the more than 47 million people with dementia globally, she spoke at the UN World Health Organization's First Ministerial Conference on Dementia in Geneva in March 2015. She is also a member of the World Dementia Council and board member of Alzheimer's Disease International. Kate volunteers on numerous consumer and working groups, including having been a member of the Dementia Working Group of The International Consortium for Health Outcomes Measurement (ICHOM) and working on the Standard Set for Dementia, released in 2016.

In 2015 Kate was winner of the Dementia Leader, University of Stirling International Dementia Awards 2015, winner of the National Disability Award as one of two emerging leaders in disability awareness, winner of the Bethanie Education medal, and a SA Finalist, Australian of The Year Awards 2016. Kate feels her most important work to date, is her role in DAI, which directly connects and supports people with dementia through online support groups around the world to live better, more connected lives. Helping others and working on ways to make the world a better place is her real drive. Kate's first book, *What the hell happened to my brain?: Living beyond dementia* was released in January 2016. She is a 'glass half full' type of girl, and when it seems empty, works hard to fill it up.

Lee-Fay Low is Associate Professor for Ageing and Health, University of Sydney. Her first job when she left university was as a home care worker for people with dementia. She is now a registered psychologist who has been conducting research in dementia for 16 years and has published over 80 research articles. Her research has included epidemiological studies looking at risk factors for dementia, qualitative interviews and focus groups to understand how people with dementia and their care partners manage dementia, and intervention studies to improve care. Her research includes working in the home care and residential aged care sector. Lee-Fay also volunteers on numerous committees, though not as many as Kate! Lee-Fay is passionate about improving the lives of people with dementia and their care partners. Her first book *Live and Laugh with Dementia* was on meaningful activities for people with dementia. She likes to look on the bright side of life.

Foreword

Dementia is never one person's illness. Its ripples spread wide, enveloping family, touching friends and bumping up against professional services and care. Dementia can be cruel — hard for those affected and sometimes even harder for care partners. When Alzheimer's and other dementia came out of the cupboard in the late 1970s, lots of advice was provided for carers or caregivers (as care partners are commonly called) with support groups internationally focusing on them. In the last decade the voice of people with dementia is now being heard more clearly. In the past, the emphasis was on the negative aspects, which of course exist. Now we are hearing about how to live with the positive.

This book is unique! It stands out from the thousands of books that have been published on dementia. It is told from the viewpoint of a person who has been living successfully with dementia and a researcher interested in living well in later life and with dementia.

When Kate Swaffer was diagnosed with dementia before her fiftieth birthday, she eventually rejected the prevailing dogma of Prescribed Disengagement®. She prescribed her own formula of engagement which includes writing — this book is just one of her contributions — studying for her PhD and advocating. And when Kate is not travelling to Geneva to talk to the United Nations or attending a conference, she is a wife and a person who wants to enjoy life. In living with dementia, Kate has developed strategies on how to cope with her disAbilities. We can all benefit by learning from her.

Associate Professor Lee-Fay Low has a wealth of experience working first as a nursing assistant in home care, as a clinical psychologist and as an academic researching dementia. Lee-Fay is creative and empathic. She is on a mission to put fun back into life for seniors and especially for people with dementia. It was Lee-Fay who led the SMILE study, which demonstrated that humour therapy could reduce agitation and improve depression and quality of life for residents of nursing homes who had dementia and were rated as behaviourally disturbed. It was Lee-Fay who spearheaded a dance intervention in nursing homes. Lee-Fay also conceived and evaluated a program for community workers to positively engage older people receiving community care.

With such a dynamic duo of authors you can expect a book that is constructive and upbeat. But it's not Pollyanna! It's realistic and tells it as it is. The difference with this book is that Kate and Lee-Fay offer strategies and solutions. Their account is practical. It takes the reader step-by-step through the basics and then outlines different issues from diagnosis to legal issues to incontinence. You, the reader, will learn about the differences between the different types of dementia, Alzheimer's, Lewy body disease and frontal lobe dementia. You may have had questions about the different drugs for Alzheimer's and the latest 'miracle cures' that regularly appear in the media. Does coconut oil work? What are the scams? Does exercise help? Does computer cognitive training work beyond the computer? What is the best diet? When should I arrange Enduring Power of Attorney? How is Power of Attorney different to Guardianship? Are pets good for you?

Dementia requires a partnership over the long haul between persons living with dementia and their care partner, family and friends, doctors, nurses, community services, residential care and sometimes palliative care. Swaffer and Low describe what services are available. Currently, services are set up to be reactive, only coming into play in response to problems or crises. I have long advocated for a system of key workers, who would guide the person with dementia and their care partner through the complex and often bewildering maze of services. Unfortunately, we do not have such a system; yet, this book is a personal guide on how to face the challenges that the ever-changing face of dementia presents over time.

I particularly liked the chapter on Living with Dementia. Communication is so important to how couples relate generally; in dementia it's critical. There is a table in which Kate and Lee-Fay describe a care partner's communications and actions and the reactions of the spouse with dementia and how these could have been handled better.

The book does not shy away from the sensitive issues that so often are avoided — all focusing on the viewpoint of the person with dementia. You and your care partner will be interested to read about the right to sexual desire and relationships, how a person with dementia and the person's care partner handle the transition from driving, how to compensate for declining competency when still working, how to handle holidays and how to manage Christmas and family celebrations. And what if you become irritated with your care partner and your care partner becomes irritated with you? Kate and Lee-Fay beautifully describe dilemmas that arise.

This book is an affirmation that dementia is a word not a sentence. A diagnosis is the beginning of a new phase, one that most of us fear, but one that can be met and challenged. There is so much that we — people with dementia, family care partners, friends, or aged care and health workers — can all do to maximise a positive life for many years.

Professor Henry Brodaty AO MB BS MD DSc FRACP FRANZCP

Acknowledgements

We wish to acknowledge the vast number of people who gave up some of their precious time to share their professional and personal experiences of dementia with us. You have not all been quoted, but our conversations, whether in person, in a zoom room, by phone or by email, have informed this book significantly. As the authors, we only have our own experiences and perspectives, and as Professor Tom Kitwood famously said, 'If you have met one person with dementia, you have done just that. You have met ONE person with dementia.' Therefore, you have helped inform the many stories of dementia, and we feel privileged you have so willingly opened your hearts.

We talked to people living with a diagnosis, family members and care partners, husbands or wives who have or are still supporting someone with dementia, but who still prefer to call themselves husbands or wives, and some who are also comfortable with being called a carer. We've spoken to professionals, including medical doctors, speech pathologists, psychologists, psychiatrists, occupational therapists, grief counsellors, and other allied health professionals. We have talked to people working in advocacy organisations and to service providers. The professionals we talked with were mostly extraordinary in their desire to support people with dementia and their families.

The real stories you have so willingly shared with us have ensured we could bring a greater depth into our book of the experience of living with dementia, or of supporting someone with dementia, and it is those individuals we have quite specifically written this book for. There are quite literally hundreds of books and research articles for professionals, but very few books or resources that have covered most things a family or individual will want to know in one place, and will likely face if dementia enters their personal world. Without your stories, we could not have come even remotely close to achieving this book, and we salute you for your honesty.

Sharing from the heart comes with an emotional cost, and many of you have shared from unfathomable depths inside your hearts, with very personal and often painful contributions of your experience and personal worlds. Thank you. We hope you know it will help others facing what you are already going through, or have been through. You have made not only a difference to this book; you will make a significant contribution to improving the lives and experiences of those who read this book.

We are indebted to you all.

Thank you.

Kate Swaffer and Lee-Fay Low

We wish to acknowledge the traditional owners of country throughout Australia, and their continuing connection to land, sea and community. We pay our respects to them and their cultures, and to elders both past, present and emerging.

CONTENTS

Introduction

No one gives you a handbook or simple guide with everything you need to know when you or someone you love, or may have to support, is diagnosed with dementia. There is so much that you don't get told, either at the time of the diagnosis, or following it. Doctors have very limited amounts of time, and our funding system and health care system is not set up to support those who need lots of time to absorb the diagnosis.

To find more than basic information on dementia you have to read many fact sheets or help sheets and, quite literally, learn to scour the internet. There is not much information for people with dementia about how to live well, or with and beyond dementia. In this book we suggest proactive strategies for living with dementia, rather than only dying from it. We show that being diagnosed with dementia does not have to be the most dreaded experience of them all. Whilst people with dementia are changing, we are still here, and can live a better life than the ones portrayed most often in the media. We talk about people with dementia having disAbilities (with the focus on their Abilities), with the same human rights as others, and capabilities to be rehabilitated and supported to continue living good lives.

Most people learn about how to manage dementia through experience, and often feel like they make many mistakes that could have been avoided if they had more information in the early days. In this book we have brought together a collection of the lived experiences of people with dementia and their care partners who have faced a diagnosis of dementia before you. We've collated tips and strategies from many people we've spoken with as well as our own experience on living with dementia, as well as the latest research evidence.

There are few published guides on how to be a care partner of a person with dementia. There are many guides for 'carers' or 'caregivers' — with the emphasis on providing care. Our emphasis is on providing information that will help families and friends to be partners in care with someone with dementia, and enablers in living well with dementia, and so we use the phrase 'care partner' rather than carer or caregiver.

There are many issues and situations you will not think about until it happens to you, or, unless someone tells you. For example, how do you cope emotionally when your dementia causes you to make mistakes and you feel your abilities slipping away? How will you react if people start talking about you like you're not there because you have dementia? For many, this happens at the point of diagnosis. What will you do when going out becomes more difficult? As a care partner, how will you talk to the person with dementia about their unsafe driving? How will it feel to put your husband of 62 or even 80 years into a nursing home? Will it feel like an enforced 'divorce'? How will you react when your wife forgets she is married to you and starts a relationship with another man, or even another woman? We share how others have reacted and managed in these situations. We give you different voices from varying perspectives; the voices of someone with dementia, their spouse, their parent, their child, their friends.

If you have been diagnosed with a dementia, or are a care partner for someone with dementia, you may have been told it will be a tough gig, and that you will have some difficult times ahead of you. Hardly anyone will tell you that you will also experience some of the most beautiful and joyous moments of your life, and there can be some incredibly positive personal growth in the experience for all involved.

Sometimes you will want to sit in a corner and cry, other days something might seem really funny, but then you might wonder, 'Is it okay to laugh when it is because of something that has happened due to dementia?' Before a diagnosis of dementia, you might do something 'stupid' and you would laugh about it, so why not laugh about some of the things that happen when you have dementia, or are supporting a person with dementia. If you don't laugh, some days you might never stop crying.

For example, a few years ago, Kate's husband picked her up to drop her off to a meeting she was going to and halfway there asked where she needed to go. She'd forgotten to bring the address with her, so replied, 'Well, actually, I have no idea!' They both could have gotten angry or upset by this — it was wasting his time, she was going to be late to the meeting — but instead, they laughed so hard he had to pull over to avoid an accident. It was better for them both to see the funny side of it. All too often, people seem afraid to have fun with dementia.

The political, funding and policy landscape for dementia is constantly changing in Australia. By the time you read this, you may find that some of the resources or services we suggest may no longer be available or may need to be accessed differently. The states and territories also differ in how and what they provide. Even if you can't access the particular resource we suggest, you will know that such things are available and you can search for an alternative. We know that many of you will go straight to Dr Google, in fact, Google searches in your state are often the best way to find up-to-date information on services. For example: 'dementia support groups in NSW' or 'dementia care in SA'.

In this book, we may have missed things out that will support you, but we have worked hard to add in as many things as we can humanly think of. Certainly, if we miss something out that has been a concern for you, we would appreciate hearing from you for the next edition, if we are lucky enough to ever have the opportunity or need to write one.

If you're reading this book, you are probably experiencing dementia personally, either as a person diagnosed with dementia, or a care partner or supporter, or a family member or friend of someone who has been diagnosed with dementia. You may also just be worried about whether you might have dementia. We hope you find this book useful, and we hope it gives you hope that you can keep living a good life. We hope it gives you confidence to stay active, to speak up for yourself, or speak up for your family member or friend with dementia, and to ask for help, access services and fight for your or their rights.

There is a psychological theory that to flourish in life we need to experience three positive emotions for every one negative emotion. We want this book to inspire more people with dementia and their care partners to flourish. Ahead of you there will be difficult, exhausting and sad times, but rather than focus only on the negatives, we hope you will find ways to make sure that there are also enjoyable, happy, fulfilling, and meaningful times and also some moments of pure joy.

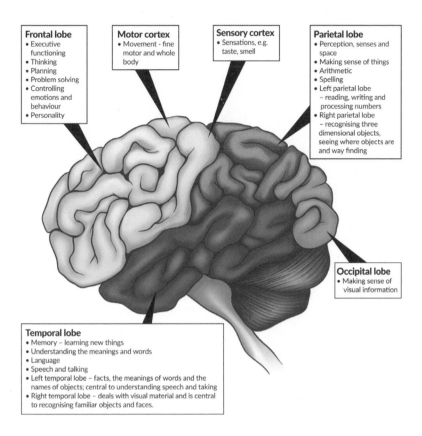

Frontal lobe
- Executive functioning
- Thinking
- Planning
- Problem solving
- Controlling emotions and behaviour
- Personality

Motor cortex
- Movement - fine motor and whole body

Sensory cortex
- Sensations, e.g. taste, smell

Parietal lobe
- Perception, senses and space
- Making sense of things
- Arithmetic
- Spelling
- Left parietal lobe – reading, writing and processing numbers
- Right parietal lobe – recognising three dimensional objects, seeing where objects are and way finding

Occipital lobe
- Making sense of visual information

Temporal lobe
- Memory – learning new things
- Understanding the meanings and words
- Language
- Speech and talking
- Left temporal lobe – facts, the meanings of words and the names of objects; central to understanding speech and taking
- Right temporal lobe – deals with visual material and is central to recognising familiar objects and faces.

Chapter 1

THE PROCESS OF BEING TESTED AND GETTING A DIAGNOSIS

What is dementia?

One of the most common questions we get asked is: what is the difference between Alzheimer's disease and dementia?

The word dementia is an umbrella term for almost 130 types or causes of a dementia, including Alzheimer's disease. Examples of umbrella terms are 'car' or 'fruit'. There are many types of cars, both by manufacturer (e.g. Toyota, Ford, Audi) and model (e.g. Toyota Corolla). There are also many types of fruit (e.g. apples, oranges, pineapples) and varieties of those fruits (e.g. Granny Smith apples, Valencia oranges). In the same way, dementia is an umbrella term for a group of diseases where the brain deteriorates (neurodegenerative diseases). Alzheimer's disease is the most common type of dementia, but other common forms are vascular dementia, Lewy Body dementia and frontotemporal dementia. Within the common forms of dementia there are also subtypes. For instance, there are several types of frontotemporal dementia including a frontotemporal dementia behavioural variant, frontotemporal dementia semantic variant and frontotemporal dementia progressive primary aphasia.

In our interviews, some people with dementia indicated their type of dementia by saying; 'I've got YOD.' This is not accurate, since YOD is the acronym for Younger Onset Dementia (meaning when a person is diagnosed under the age of 65), however, a person with YOD can have Alzheimer's disease, Vascular dementia or any of the other types of dementia.

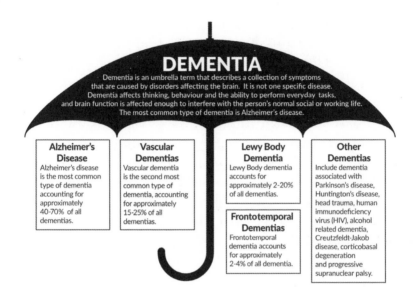

DEMENTIA

Dementia is an umbrella term that describes a collection of symptoms that are caused by disorders affecting the brain. It is not one specific disease. Dementia affects thinking, behaviour and the ability to perform everyday tasks, and brain function is affected enough to interfere with the person's normal social or working life. The most common type of dementia is Alzheimer's disease.

Alzheimer's Disease
Alzheimer's disease is the most common type of dementia accounting for approximately 40-70% of all dementias.

Vascular Dementias
Vascular dementia is the second most common type of dementia, accounting for approximately 15-25% of all dementias.

Lewy Body Dementia
Lewy Body dementia accounts for approximately 2-20% of all dementias.

Frontotemporal Dementias
Frontotemporal dementia accounts for approximately 2-4% of all dementia.

Other Dementias
Include dementia associated with Parkinson's disease, Huntington's disease, head trauma, human immunodeficiency virus (HIV), alcohol related dementia, Creutzfeldt-Jakob disease, corticobasal degeneration and progressive supranuclear palsy.

The difference between dementia and ageing

For many years it was thought that memory loss was nothing more than the hardening of the arteries experienced by most people during the natural ageing process. Often called 'senility', it was common to equate the behaviours of someone with dementia with 'old age senility', causing erratic or odd behaviour. Many people still believe that dementia is a normal part of ageing; however, it is not. You could live to a very old age and still not have dementia. The oldest documented woman in the world, Jeanne Calment, did not have dementia when she passed away at age 122 years. Half of people aged over 100 years don't have dementia.

What is the difference between dementia and normal memory loss with ageing?

Our brains grow from childhood into our early twenties. From our forties, the brain starts to shrink very slowly both because of loss of neurons (brain cells) and connections between these cells. It is around this time that we start to notice changes in our memory. As we age, blood flow to our brain also decreases. The temporal and frontal lobes seem to be more affected by ageing than other parts of the brain. The temporal lobe is responsible for memory and the frontal lobes for 'executive function'— learning new things, organising and planning.

Memory for words, facts and concepts (e.g. the capital of Germany — we call this type of memory semantic memory) and on how to do things (e.g. how to drive a car — we call this type of memory procedural memory) does not decline much with ageing. Memory for the specific sequence of events that have happened (e.g. where did I spend my fortieth birthday and who was there with me — we call this type of memory episodic memory) declines with age. As the brain ages it is not unusual to forget the name of someone, particularly if you haven't seen him or her for some time. Ageing can make it difficult to remember the right word when speaking or writing, or hard to remember the name of an object that isn't used often.

With older age, it takes longer to learn new skills or accept new ideas. It may take longer to react to things since reflexes slow down with the ageing process.

All these changes are normal parts of ageing, and not necessarily a sign that someone has dementia. The difference between normal ageing and dementia is the extent of the memory and thinking difficulties and how they interfere with the person's day-to-day life — and this is what makes it particularly difficult to distinguish normal ageing from the early signs of dementia.

Who can give a diagnosis of dementia?

Typically, dementia is diagnosed by a doctor, either a general practitioner or specialist (usually a neurologist, geriatrician or psychogeriatrician), though another health professional can also make the diagnosis. Australian general practitioners are not always confident in diagnosing dementia, so when symptoms are milder and are harder to distinguish from normal ageing, or the person is younger (under the age of 65) they are often sent to a specialist for diagnosis. General practitioners are more likely to make the diagnosis themselves if the symptoms are more severe and the person is older.

How long does it take to get a diagnosis?

In Australia, symptoms of dementia are noticed by families an average of 1.9 years before they discuss them with a doctor, and there is an average of 3.1 years between noticing symptoms and obtaining a firm diagnosis of dementia. Time to diagnosis is affected by how much insight the person and their family have into the symptoms and how much the symptoms impact on the person's life, the knowledge and attitudes the first health professional they talk to (usually their general practitioner) has about dementia and access to specialist services. People who have had higher cognitive abilities (a higher IQ) may more easily compensate for the cognitive changes in the earlier stage, and this may also make it more difficult to get a diagnosis as, often, previous cognitive abilities are not considered.

Time to diagnosis is also affected by how typical the person's presentation is. It may take longer, or more health practitioner visits before diagnosis, for rarer or unusual forms of dementia (i.e. if memory difficulties are not prominent) or for dementia in younger people (i.e. under the age of 65). Some general practitioners and other medical professionals used to think that there was no point in diagnosing dementia as there is little they can do, or were afraid that giving someone a diagnosis of dementia would ruin their relationship with them — some doctors may still think this way. For some people, their doctor may suspect they have dementia but not offer to investigate further. If you are worried about cognitive changes and this happens to you (many have told us it happened to them), then do seek the advice of another medical practitioner, or insist on a referral to a memory clinic or specialist such as a neurologist or geriatrician.

For people over 65, dementia is now the most feared disease, more feared than cancer and, therefore, many older people put off seeking a diagnosis, or even telling their general practitioner they have concerns. Some people are afraid of acknowledging that something is wrong and others are worried about the stigma surrounding dementia in the community and about being embarrassed, laughed at, or ignored by acquaintances and friends.

We've met many families where the person with dementia has refused to see a medical professional, despite being strongly urged to do so by their close family and friends. While we believe that obtaining a diagnosis and knowing what is wrong is better than not knowing, there is no research evidence yet to suggest that people who are diagnosed earlier in the course of the disease do better over time. We believe strongly that people with dementia should be supported and enabled to maintain control of their lives, and this includes not 'forcing' them to obtain a formal diagnosis.

Most of the actions that we describe in this book (e.g. staying active) don't require a formal diagnosis of dementia.

How is dementia diagnosed?

In a nutshell, dementia is diagnosed if the person is declining in memory and other thinking processes, this decline impacts on how they live their day-to-day life, and there is no other explanation for the symptoms.

The formal criteria for a diagnosis of dementia, irrespective of type, according to the American National Institutes of Health and Alzheimer's Association, require that for a person to be diagnosed with **probable or possible** dementia:

---

1. There are changes in memory and thinking (known as cognition) or changes in behaviour, which interfere with the person's ability to work or perform their usual activities.

---

2. The changes are declines in the person's **usual** abilities, not things they have always had trouble with. The person doesn't need to be performing more poorly than others their age.

So, if the person has always had a poor memory, or trouble reading maps, and this has gotten worse similarly to others their own age, it is not considered a decline which would meet criteria for a diagnosis of dementia. If a person has been exceptional in an area (e.g. a lifetime working as a chartered accountant) and now reports difficulty completing a tax return, this would be considered a decline even if testing suggests that numeracy is similar to others. Being able to judge whether a person has declined makes it more difficult to diagnose early dementia in people who were of high intelligence or, conversely, who had learning difficulties before the dementia.

---

3. The changes are not explained by delirium or mental illness.

Some of the symptoms of delirium, depression, anxiety, post-traumatic stress disorder (PTSD) and other mental illnesses are similar to dementia and sometimes delirium and depression are referred to as 'pseudo dementias'. These conditions have well-established treatments, which can completely reverse the symptoms, or improve them. Therefore, before being able to diagnose dementia, the doctor will check to see if the person has delirium, depression, anxiety or another major mental illness. If the person does have one or more of these conditions the doctor will treat the other conditions to see if the symptoms have been caused by these conditions. If the symptoms remain after the conditions have been treated, then the person may have dementia. Untreated or unresolved grief may also be the cause of cognitive changes, and, with loss and grief counselling, the cognitive changes may also be resolved. This is why later in the book we recommend grief and loss counselling for people diagnosed with dementia, as unresolved grief following a diagnosis may make the symptoms of dementia seem worse or the person's decline appear more rapid.

Doctors will also try and rule out physical conditions, which may cause the changes in memory and thinking. Blood tests are often done as part of the investigations to look for medical conditions such as low Vitamin B12 and folate levels and poor thyroid function, which may cause the symptoms. Urine tests and a chest X-ray may be undertaken, again to rule out other physical causes.

---

4. Changes in memory and thinking are established by asking the person suspected of having dementia, and a family member or friend who knows them well, to reveal the history of their symptoms (this is known as a case history), AND by objectively

testing cognition. The case history is important in establishing the changes that have been happening.

At the minimum, a short cognitive screening test will be conducted. The most commonly used test is the mini-mental state examination (MMSE) which includes items such as the current day and date, and counting backwards from 100 in sevens. A perfect score on the MMSE is 30/30, and a score of 23 or less suggests possible cognitive impairment. The test is not always accurate in picking up dementia, as some people with dementia get perfect scores on the MMSE, and it is also common for people without dementia to score between 27 and 29.

If the symptom history and screening test is inconclusive in establishing whether there are changes in memory or thinking, then neuropsychological assessment may be conducted. This typically involves two–three hours of memory and thinking tests conducted by a psychologist or neuropsychologist. Tests include those of memory for word and number lists and stories, memory for visual patterns, planning (such as when copying a picture) and different kinds of problem solving such as figuring out the 'rules' of a problem and adapting when the rules change without explanation.

Most neuropsychological tests are designed to test all levels of ability — this means that it is nearly impossible to get perfect scores on most tests, and many people get at least some answers wrong. Psychologists are trained to not tell those being tested if they got items right or wrong, but test subjects can feel strange getting neutral feedback. They also do tests to ensure a person is not faking poor performance. Many people find neuropsychological testing stressful, frustrating, or depressing.

---

5. The declines in cognition have to be in at least two areas:

i. memory (e.g. frequently losing things, forgetting events, getting lost)

ii. problem solving (e.g. poor decision-making, not being able to handle finances)

iii. processing of visual information (e.g. not being able to read a map, not being able to recognise familiar people or common objects)

iv. ability to use language (e.g. forgetting common words, trouble with writing or reading), and

v. changes in personality, behaviour or comportment (e.g. losing interest in things she previously enjoyed, being more withdrawn, more irritable or more impulsive).

A routine part of investigations are brain scans. Usually this is a computerised tomography or CT scan. This is not necessary to diagnose dementia, but helps clinicians increase the certainty of their diagnosis and give information on the subtype of dementia. A clinician will check the scan for damage and deterioration, such as dead areas of brain, suggesting strokes or mini strokes, and areas where there is atrophy or shrinking of the brain (indicated by bigger than expected spaces within the brain or between the brain and the skull cavity). Sometimes more sensitive scans such as a magnetic resonance imaging (MRI) or a positron emission tomography (PET) scan may also be done.

It is not possible to diagnose dementia by looking at a scan alone, people who have what may look to a radiologist like an 'abnormal' scan may not have any symptoms of dementia, and conversely people who have symptoms of dementia may have changes on their scans which are consistent with their age.

Diagnosing different subtypes of dementia

Diagnosing the subtype of dementia is more difficult for clinicians than deciding whether the person has dementia or not. A neurological examination, brain scans and neuropsychological test results all contribute to helping decide what type of dementia the person may have. While the diagnostic criteria try to make clear-cut distinctions between different types of dementia, we often see 'mixed' cases — most commonly mixed Alzheimer's disease with vascular dementia, but also other combinations.

Diagnostic criteria for Alzheimer's disease

To be diagnosed with possible Alzheimer's disease the person must:

---

1. Meet criteria for dementia.

---

2. Have gradual onset of symptoms over months to years, not sudden over hours or days.

---

3. Have a clear history of decline in cognition.

---

4. Based on the symptom history and cognitive testing there could be clear impairments in one of the following:

i. short-term memory i.e. in learning and recalling new information as well (this is the most common presentation in Alzheimer's disease); or

ii. language, including trouble word-finding; or

iii. processing of visual information i.e. recognising familiar people or objects; or

iv. reasoning, judgement and problem solving; may be more impulsive and less decisive (clinicians refer to these as executive or higher-order functions of the brain).

---

5. Have impairments on another area of cognitive functioning.

---

6. NOT show symptoms or evidence based on history or testing of which suggests another type of dementia, another active neurological disease, or a non-neurological medical condition or medication that could have a substantial effect on cognition.

Diagnostic criteria for vascular dementia

To be diagnosed with possible vascular dementia, the person must:

1. Meet the general diagnostic criteria for dementia.

2. Show signs of cerebrovascular disease (disease to the blood circulation of the brain) on neurological testing and in a brain scan.

3. Have a history suggesting that the symptoms of dementia and the cerebrovascular disease are related, such as onset of dementia within three months of a stroke, or abrupt, stepwise progression or fluctuating cognitive symptoms. There may be great variability in symptoms depending on location of brain damage.

Diagnostic criteria for dementia with Lewy bodies

To be diagnosed with possible dementia with Lewy bodies, the person must:

1. Meet the general diagnostic criteria for dementia.

2. Have one or more of the following:

    i. fluctuating cognition, particularly variations in attention and alertness;

    ii. recurring visual hallucinations (seeing things that aren't really there);

    iii. Parkinsonism symptoms such as slowness and decrease in the normal range in movement, difficulty initiating movements, rigidity, resting tremor;

    iv. REM sleep behaviour disorder;

v. Severe sensitivity to the medication class of neuroleptics; or

vi. Low dopamine transporter uptake in basal ganglia demonstrated by SPECT or PET imaging.

Diagnostic criteria for frontotemporal dementia

To be diagnosed with possible frontotemporal dementia the person must:

1. Meet diagnostic criteria for dementia.

2. The behavioural and cognitive symptoms started with either:

i. Early and ongoing changes in personality, such as difficulty in controlling own behaviour; or loss of drive, interest or initiative or loss of sympathy or empathy; repetitive or compulsive behaviours such as clapping, tapping, counting, checking and rechecking; eating more — sweets, fatty foods, bingeing, alcohol or cigarettes or eating inedible objects (this would suggest behavioural variant frontotemporal dementia);

ii. Early and ongoing change in language, such as having trouble expressing themselves, a great deal of trouble finding the right word, or not understanding the meanings of words (this would suggest semantic variant frontotemporal dementia).

Aphasia is a form of cognitive impairment that involves progressive loss of language function.

The following is a short piece to help someone with a dementia that causes them to have aphasia or to help families and care partners be more supportive and understanding. If you search YouTube, you will find others like this, on symptoms other than aphasia, and many people with dementia, sharing their lived experiences.

Understanding Aphasia: Imagine life without words

Aphasia is a complex condition that varies in every individual. Some have difficulty understanding speech; some find it hard to talk, while others have difficulty reading and writing. In cases of severe aphasia all these four modes of communicating can be significantly affected.

———

Millions of people are diagnosed with aphasia around the world, largely due to a 30% prevalence in stroke survivors, but how much do we really understand the impact on people's lives? What can we do to improve the quality of life for people with aphasia? It's time that this population has a voice. It starts with awareness, breaking down misconceptions. It needs to conclude with a challenge of how we can better support people with aphasia, so they can feel connected and integrated into their communities.

———

The video comes in a short and extended version, and the producers have made it available publicly here https://www. youtube.com/watch?v=OGyOKItHS9Y to educate others, particularly in the health sector, where the care can only be enhanced by good communication. It will be helpful for families and care partners of a person with dementia to watch it as well.

Unintended consequences of the diagnosis process

Diagnostic criteria for dementia require doctors to show that the person has declined and has deficits — this means that doctors test for what the person can't do, and the abilities that the person has 'lost'.

Unfortunately, this then carries over to how the person is cared for after the diagnosis — the person is seen as a set of 'deficits' and 'losses' rather than as someone with strengths and abilities capable of having an impact in the world (see Chapter 2 for more on Prescribed Disengagement).

The fact that diagnosing dementia is complex, and can take a long time, means people with dementia and their families often face a prolonged period of uncertainty and worrying about what is wrong. After the effort and build up to getting a diagnosis, it is sometimes deflating to then be given an information brochure rather than ongoing support. Some people we interviewed reported they were given no information at all at the time of diagnosis, not even a brochure about dementia or where to go for support.

When asked what information she would have liked to have been given after her family member was given the diagnosis, one person said:

> *I wanted a human being,* one *person I could talk to, someone to support me and Mum. Every person diagnosed with dementia should have access to a case worker for whatever level of intensity they require, from diagnosis to death. DON'T give me a pamphlet or a webpage. This is a matter for talking about really important things between human beings.*

Is it possible that the diagnosis is wrong?

Clinicians take giving someone a diagnosis of dementia very seriously. There are implications that receiving such a diagnosis has on how people choose to live their lives, how they see themselves, and how others see them. Most clinicians we know tend to err on the side of caution and will not give the diagnosis unless they are relatively certain that the person has dementia. So almost all people diagnosed as having dementia will probably have dementia. However, we have known of a handful of cases where the diagnosis was incorrect and the person over time did not have dementia.

Currently, the only way to make a definite diagnosis of any type of dementia is through a postmortem brain autopsy. Kate Swaffer has regularly said she is not quite ready for that type of confirmation! Brain scanning technology is improving so that in the future it will be possible to get a brain scan to definitively show that there is Alzheimer's Disease pathology (i.e. beta amyloid) in the brain. At the moment there are only a few radiology laboratories in Australia able to offer these scans and they are expensive.

I've been diagnosed with mild cognitive impairment — what does this mean?

A diagnosis of Mild Cognitive Impairment (MCI) is given to people who don't have 'normal' memory and thinking but do not meet the criteria for dementia — either because they only have impairments in one area of cognition, or because the difficulties do not interfere with their day-to-day life. Mild cognitive impairment is thought of as a stage between normal ageing and dementia. People who have mild cognitive impairment are more likely to go on to develop dementia, but this will not necessarily happen. If you've been diagnosed with mild cognitive impairment, it is likely that the doctor will schedule you to return for retesting in six months or a year. There is a lot of research happening involving people with mild cognitive impairment, as it is thought that intervening in this group may prevent or delay the onset of dementia.

How common is dementia?

The prevalence of dementia increases with age and about doubles with every ten years of age. Between 0.054% and 0.068% of people aged between 30 and 65 have dementia. In contrast, according to the Alzheimer's Australia, 1 in 10 people over the age of 65 have dementia.

How many people have dementia?

Dementia currently affects more than 47.5 million people globally. One person is newly diagnosed with dementia every 3.2 seconds somewhere in the world, equating to 7.7 million new cases per year[1]. In Australia, there are currently 353,800 people diagnosed with dementia, meaning that each week in Australia, there are more than 1,800 new cases of dementia, or approximately one person diagnosed every six minutes[2]. It is currently the second highest cause of death in Australia, and the most feared disease for people over the age of 65, higher than cancer. Dementia is the biggest

---

1 *World Health Organization,* Dementia Fact Sheet 362, *2015http://www.who. int/mediacentre/factsheets/fs362/en*

2 *Alzheimer's Australia,* Key Facts and Statistics For Media: Key Facts and Statistics *2016 https://fightdementia.org.au/national/media/key-facts-and-statistics*

health and social challenge facing the developed and developing world. As the prevalence of dementia increases with age, this number will continue to rise as the average age of the population rises. Dementia is one of the major causes of disability and dependency.

Does it really matter what type of dementia I have?

In people aged over 65, Alzheimer's disease is the most common form of dementia, estimated at between 40 and 75% of cases. Vascular dementia accounts for between 15 and 25% of cases, frontotemporal dementia between 2 and 4% of cases, Lewy body dementia between 2 and 20%, and mixed dementia between 10 and 20%.

Since it is the most common, Alzheimer's disease is also the stereotypical form of dementia. If your symptoms differ from a traditional Alzheimer's profile, health practitioners may take longer to recognise your symptoms, may be surprised by them, and may not know how to help manage them. For instance, aged care staff may not realise that the strong preference for sweet foods is a symptom of frontotemporal dementia and a resident may put on weight in an unhealthy way. Treatments available according to dementia subtype are discussed in Chapter 4.

Are my children going to get dementia?

Genetically inherited forms of dementia are very rare, only about 1–2% of all cases of dementia are caused by genes — meaning that if you have the gene you are certain to eventually develop dementia if you live long enough. People who have genetically determined dementia usually start showing symptoms when they are younger, before the age of 65.

If you and many (i.e. a third or half) of your first degree relatives have similar dementias which started before the age of 65, then you may have a genetically inherited form. Speak to your doctor if this is the case. Genetic testing for dementia is not readily available, and it is a big decision to get tested.

I have a very strong family history of dementia; it is very likely that I carry the gene for Alzheimer's. This has more poignancy for me due to my professional understanding of what dementia can entail for someone. I have seen, in my 25 years as a doctor, the effects dementia has on family, friends, people with the diagnosis and their carers. I am scared, I will not deny that, I do not want to lose what I hold in my head. I am going to go on a journey to discover if I have the gene for Alzheimer's and I am not going to bury my head in the sand and hope for the best. I am going to learn how to improve my memory and the workings of my brain. - A medical doctor

For non-genetically inherited dementias, genes may still contribute to the risk of getting dementia. If you're reading this and have dementia, your children may be of higher risk than someone whose parent doesn't have dementia. However, this doesn't mean that they will definitely get dementia.

Could I have done something to avoid getting dementia? As a care partner can I do something to avoid getting dementia myself?

We don't know what causes most cases of dementia. In the last 20 years, research has identified many risk factors associated with dementia. It's impossible to eliminate every single one; after all we can't avoid ageing, which is the most significant risk.

Medical conditions such as diabetes, stroke, heart problems, as well as high blood pressure, high cholesterol and obesity in mid-life, are all known to increase the risk of both Alzheimer's disease and vascular dementia, and everyone can reduce their risk by keeping these under control.

Depression is also a probable risk factor for dementia, therefore, getting it treated early is important.

Isolation is also another risk factor for dementia, so supporting anyone who is living alone to engage and socialise more is helpful.

Risk reduction for dementia

We now know that people who adopt a healthy lifestyle, especially from mid-life onwards, are less likely to develop some dementias. This means taking regular physical exercise and keeping to a healthy weight, not smoking, eating a healthy balanced diet and drinking only in moderation. Leading an active lifestyle that combines regular physical, social and mental activity will help to lower risk.

Alzheimer's Australia have a website Your Brain Matters[3], which lists five steps to care for your brain and reduce your risk of dementia:

---

1. Step One: Look after your heart — this includes making sure that you have treated your high blood pressure, high cholesterol, type 2 diabetes and obesity, and don't smoke.

---

2. Step Two: Be physically active — follow the national physical activity guidelines (see Chapter 3 for these).

---

3. Step Three: Mentally challenge your brain.

---

4. Step Four: Follow a healthy diet — follow the national dietary guidelines (see Chapter 3 for these too!).

---

5. Step Five: Enjoy social activity.

If you don't have dementia, and even if you do have a diagnosis, we recommend you review your health and lifestyle, in the same way we are all advised to do this for our overall health.

---

3 *Alzheimer's Australia http://yourbrainmatters.org.au*

Chapter 2

WHEN FIRST DIAGNOSED— FEELINGS AND PRESCRIBED DISENGAGEMENT®

Responses to a diagnosis

Many report that getting a diagnosis of dementia is often a very demanding and lengthy experience, and a long, painful, difficult period of their life. Many also report the experience of being told they or a family member has dementia is less than optimal.

One daughter said:

> We went to the memory clinic, which was really just a geriatrician and all they could offer mum was access to medication. There was absolutely nothing else on offer. No counsellor, no social worker, no-one. Nothing. I was left to deal with everything myself. The geriatrician at the memory clinic had no skills to talk with Mum, there was no understanding, no empathy, no respect. It was an awful experience and very damaging for Mum and I.

When a person is first diagnosed with a dementia, their world and their family's or supporters' worlds changes forever, and it is at this time they really need support. The impact of a diagnosis of dementia varies with each individual, but common feelings and reactions to being told you have a dementia include shock, disbelief, denial, anger, anxiety and other feelings of loss and grief. As dementia is a terminal, progressive and chronic illness, the fear of what may be ahead is also difficult, and can impact many other things. The person diagnosed is thrown into complete turmoil: 'why me?', 'surely it's not true', 'let's get a second/third opinion', and many other responses.

One person with dementia said: 'It initially felt like a death sentence to me; a dose of cruel reality that screamed 'no hope' like a neon lamp.'

Kate Swaffer wrote when first diagnosed (although it will be obvious as you read this book, that the following reaction to her being told she had dementia is not the only one she had, and her experiences of living with dementia are often now, far more positive):

> *Most days are now an effort not to just sit in a corner and cry, not to just give up or to give in to it. It requires a great amount of emotional effort to live a 'normal' existence and is truly the most demeaning and frightening experience I have had, with a feeling of wretchedness I have not felt before.*
>
> *This new place is full of hidden and impending madness, full of people already whispering behind closed doors away from my ears, trying to plan for my demise and how I and they will cope. They provide words of comfort and gentle pats on my back, meaning well but never realising it usually makes me feel like a leper, as if I am to be pitied. They are the ones who will eventually have the challenges of coping, as I will be lost in a world of inhibition and supposed joyfulness, locked out of the reality of the world and its occupants. And so, I keep asking myself am I to be the lucky one in this strange place called dementia. Perhaps so.*

Families, close friends and supporters also experience this, in a different way; in part due to the fact they may have been noticing changes in the person for some time. Coming to terms with such a diagnosis is very difficult for every person diagnosed, and also for family members and friends, especially those who are care partners for the person with dementia.

Receiving a diagnosis of dementia can also be a relief — to finally know what is causing the changes, as often the person and those close to them know something is wrong and the diagnostic process can be long and complicated.

One of the first things to do when you or someone you love and support receives a diagnosis of dementia is to learn about the particular dementia they have. This will give you a better chance of living better with the diagnosis or being a better supporter.

The daughter of someone diagnosed with dementia said:

> *For the rest of my life I will always live with the guilt of not understanding dementia and its impact on my dad. Had I known the prognosis and the trajectory, I would certainly have been able to take much better care of my dad and demonstrated my love for him more often. I would have tried to know from him more about his life and things that were important to him and would have shared both my important and not-so-important stories with him. I would have made so many more memories with my dad!*

She also said, when asked what she wanted when looking back on her experience: 'Information, information, information.'

Dr Al Power has a more positive way to view the definition of dementia, suggesting that if we view it differently, others will respond more positively to people with dementia, and people with dementia may see it as less devastating. He says,[4] 'Dementia is a shift in the way a person experiences the world around her/him.'

Loss and grief

People with dementia and their supporters benefit greatly from grief and loss counselling, not only counselling to manage the changes to personality or behaviours, but to help them with the intense loss and grief they are all facing. The loss and grief caused by a diagnosis of dementia

---

4 *GA Power,* Dementia Beyond Disease: Enhancing Well-Being, *Health Professions Press, Baltimore, 2014*

is often not considered or recognised and therefore under-treated, and is also very complicated. There is a lot in the literature about the loss and grief experienced by care partners and friends and families, in particular, on the anticipatory grief they feel and their loss and grief after someone they love has died, but very little on the loss and grief of the person with dementia.

People with dementia feel things such as a significant fear of a loss of identity, the loss of privacy and loss of friends. They fear simple things, like wondering if they will remember their children, partners, friends or other family members' faces and names. Not knowing what to call simple things you have always known the names of also causes feelings of loss and grief, as well as frustration and feelings of incompetence.

Grief can feel like a constant companion; the grief caused by being diagnosed with a dementia almost, literally, never goes away. When you lose someone or even something (e.g. a house in a bushfire) you love, eventually, you learn to live without them or it, but you do eventually get used to your life without that person or thing and learn to live beyond your grief and create a new life. Dementia grief is not like that, and can be extremely crippling; just as you get used to the loss of some function or capacity, it then gets worse, or you 'lose' some other function or capacity. Each time the person diagnosed realises they have lost more capacity or function, a renewed sense of grief for the loss appears. This can happen many times a day and most of the time other people don't see or know about it.

These losses of function or capacity, or changes to personality or behaviour, eventually may not be obvious to the person diagnosed, but the care partner sees them and is living with increasing anticipatory grief as well. However, in the earlier phases of dementia, the person diagnosed knows and feels them profoundly, but they are invisible to most others. It is these 'invisible disabilities' that may make it more difficult for others to believe someone has dementia.

It may be important, therefore, to have ongoing grief and loss counselling, in order to be able to live a good life. But it is worth remembering, the grief of these losses, caused by the deterioration of current capacity, or of a new symptom of dementia, does not go away. It won't heal either, because dementia will and does get worse, not better.

People with dementia and their care partners and families should be careful not to let the grief consume them constantly. It is important to find support, to accept the diagnosis and manage the grief well, and to find ways to put it on hold some of the time, so you can still live with joy.

Acceptance does not mean giving up or not 'fighting for your life'. Acceptance does not mean resignation. Acceptance means accepting the changes that have happened and may happen in the future, and problem solving and working around these to continue reaching goals and living life beyond a diagnosis of dementia, instead of immediately assuming the pseudo death many talk about and expect.

Nothing left in the tank

We have all experienced that feeling of having 'nothing left in the tank'. It can happen when we are working too hard, or raising kids, or studying, or trying to do all three at once. It can happen to anyone, anytime, and does not need a crisis to cause it. In this fast-paced world we are living in, some days breathing and getting out of bed seems like hard work, even without dementia.

When you are diagnosed with dementia, or supporting someone living with dementia, there will be days when you both feel there is 'nothing left in the tank'. Often, those days won't meet up, the person diagnosed might feel frustrated or like they are running on empty on a day when the care partner is okay. This is not dissimilar to shared loss; when a couple grieves the loss of a child, they rarely experience or express the same feelings on the same day. This can lead to huge frustrations and quite often anger towards each other, as the partner feeling the grief more acutely that day can think the other parent doesn't care. It is complex.

Having dementia come into your life at close proximity is truly traumatic and stressful, and we cannot stress enough how important it is to get support as soon as possible.

Get the tough emotional things done quickly, like the wills and other end of life affairs (see Chapter 5 — planning ahead), so you can get on with living and forget about them, especially if you are the person with a new diagnosis of dementia, so your family doesn't have to worry about it. They need to know what to do, and more importantly, what YOU WANT if your dementia progresses more quickly than you might expect, and you lose capacity to make those decisions for yourself. Many times, it is these types of things that become the obstacles for living beyond dementia, and that cause friction between families, friends and couples.

There will be days when you want to hide or run away. There will be days when no matter what you do as a care partner or friend of someone with dementia, their experience might appear dreadful, or they might not appreciate your effort.

There will be days as a person with dementia when you will feel deep guilt for having been the 'cause of the stress', and days when the fear of what is ahead, for both of you, feels like too much to bear.

Many days, living in the denial bubble is the only choice you will be able to make, especially when you are not coping emotionally with dementia. Perhaps even force yourself to go there occasionally. We all need 'time out' from everything, and especially from illness and impending deterioration, disease and anticipated death.

Getting support when things are going okay is helpful, as it will give you strategies to cope and manage on the really bad days. It won't take them away, but hopefully will reduce the stress when things do change or get worse.

Grief counselling, support at home, time out, respite, or a vacation can all support you on the days when there is nothing left in the tank. Plan them in advance; don't wait for the day when you can't cope, or a crisis. It is on those occasions many report that they cannot find anyone available to support them. Services are often only available from 9am–5pm; a crisis happens any time of the day or night! Even finding a way to go out with a friend for a beer or coffee may help. On the really, really, really bad days, when you don't think you can go on, if you've been getting support from someone you now have a relationship with, you can call them. This can be more helpful than calling a Helpline during your crisis and talking to a complete stranger. Also, if you have no previous relationship with that service, you might have to wait longer for support.

One care partner said; 'I am really cranky at myself for waiting for three years to ask for help. I could have so many things in place now, if I had realised how much I needed to do!'

This man's days are now more settled, but he went through, in his words, 'a very dark period', while he waded through available services, and set up some support. Accessing services is hard even when there is no crisis, but if you wait for one, the effort may be enormous.

Ms P, a lady with dementia who lives alone said, 'I so wish I had not been too proud to ask for help. Now it looks as if I can no longer care for myself, and will have to go into a home.' Since her interview for this book, she has had no choice but to go into residential care, and she is not thrilled at all.

Many think asking for help is the end of the road of independence, but in fact, it is more often the beginning of establishing more independence and control, and less stress for everyone, and may delay residential care significantly, and for many, may mean not requiring it at all. Asking for help, setting up services and support, even casual or unprofessional ones, is what will help you avoid more instances of feeling like you have 'nothing left in your tank.'

Care partner or BUB (back-up brain)

The topic of what to call the family member, partner or friend who is supporting the person with dementia is fraught with challenges. To refer to them as a carer or caregiver (or even care partner) can strip them of their other identities and other important roles, and places a 'burden' on them, and a 'burden' on the person with dementia. It takes away their control, and reduces the power of the person with dementia in their own life and choices. This can also contribute to the learned helplessness in people with dementia and 'martyrdom' of some care partners that we'll talk about later in this chapter under Prescribed Disengagement.®

Some people use terms like enabler or supporter. Kate Swaffer and her husband Peter Watt often use the term back-up brain or BUB for short, for his role in supporting and enabling her to remain independent as much as possible. If you think about how you use a back-up on your computer, the term BUB works the same way. You don't ask the back-up to do the tasks that the computer does, you only use it when the computer crashes, freezes or needs a reboot.

They think of a back-up brain as being the same as the spare hard drive in a computer, and Peter said, it empowers him to be by Kate's side, *with or alongside her*, rather than to *care for or take over from* her, a subtle but significant difference.

Offering support or assistance is key here, rather than 'caring' by doing for the other person. BUBs support and enable the person with dementia to 'do for themselves' for as long as possible, and no matter how much longer it takes is important.

With support from the Back-Up Brain, the brain (person) that is living with increasing disAbilities, can sometimes, albeit with effort, still function well for longer than many will assume possible. It also empowers the person with dementia to feel less of a failure, and less guilty about what is happening (failure, only in the sense of having to accept there are so many things one simply cannot do alone or at all any more), and removes some of the stress of being the care partner. This approach also changes the dynamics between the two parties, and is a more equitable for everyone. Having a Back-Up Brain gives people with dementia more control and say over their own lives for longer, until such time as the progression of the dementia makes it too difficult to be independent.

Dementia Myths

Some of the popular myths of dementia are not facts. If we believe in them unquestioningly, we may be supporting someone else's agenda, and also denying the person diagnosed with dementia a more positive experience.

There is no point diagnosing dementia as nothing can be done, and there is no cure

We see significant value in an early diagnosis, regardless of the fact there is no cure and no treatment for many. This is not based so much on the need to ensure end-of-life wishes are in order, but allows people to take more control of things such as their health, and to work on positive psychosocial and non-pharmacological interventions such as increasing exercise. It also gives people time to work on the activities on their bucket list!

Alzheimer's disease is not dementia

Alzheimer's disease is a type of dementia. It is more correct to say, if diagnosed with any dementia, that you have a dementia, probably of this or that type. In the same way that the words 'fruit' or 'animal' are umbrella terms, as shown in our diagram on page 17, 'dementia' is an umbrella term for around 130 different types or causes of dementia.

People with dementia are 'fading away' and 'not all there'

Even though we may be changing, people with dementia are always still all there. A person dying from terminal cancer or motor neuron disease is still all there, and so are people with dementia. We all change each and every day, and after every significant experience, and it is no different for people with dementia.

People with dementia can't communicate with you

Even in the later stages of dementia, when some may lose the ability to speak at all, people with dementia can still communicate in other ways. Others need to take the time to watch and listen to the non-verbal cues and signs of communication. Sometimes, time is all that is needed to find the words or understand someone.

A person doesn't have memory loss, therefore can't possibly have dementia

Many people become forgetful as they become older. This is common and is often not due to dementia. There are also other disorders such as depression and an underactive thyroid that can cause memory problems. Dementia is the most serious form of memory problems. Dementia includes many other symptoms besides memory loss. There are some forms of dementia where the person experiences very little memory loss until the late stages of the disease.

A person can still speak and function in public, therefore can't have dementia

This is a common misperception, especially for those people diagnosed early in the disease. Just because a person with dementia can still speak, and appears to function well in the five or 30 minutes someone spends with them, does not mean they don't have dementia. The analogy of the swan, calm and serene on the surface, paddling below the surface to stay afloat, is very apt. Often the symptoms, especially in the earlier stages of dementia are invisible to others. Also, it is not logical that the day of diagnosis, the person suddenly cannot function at all; very few people are diagnosed in the very late stage.

They don't look like they have dementia

Quite frankly, what is someone with dementia supposed to look like?! Unlike a person with cancer who might lose weight or lose their hair after treatment, people with dementia don't develop features that indicate dementia, and they are very rarely diagnosed at end stage, when it may be more obvious that they have dementia.

One man said, 'For goodness sake, am I supposed to suddenly get horns, or look stupid!'

It is fair to say that the day before a person is diagnosed no-one will say 'you look like you might have dementia', so why, the next day when one is diagnosed with it, does almost everyone say, 'but you don't look like you have dementia'?

This particular myth is reported by people diagnosed with dementia to be a major frustration and annoyance, and questioning their diagnosis is insensitive and, for many, hurtful.

People with dementia don't feel pain

Historically, we used to believe that people with dementia did not feel pain because of the effects that their illness has on the brain. We have since realised that is not so; people with dementia are just as likely as anyone else to experience pain but they cannot express it. Many patients lose the ability to talk, but even those who are coherent may struggle to find the right words to describe their discomfort. Think how frustrating that must be — you can't find the words to tell someone, 'I'm in agony', or 'This is hurting'. When Kate was working in a dementia unit, many residents said yes or no to everything, including when being questioned about pain, simply because they knew an answer was expected.

There is a growing body of research that has found that many of the symptoms often written off as just a part of the changed behaviours of dementia — agitation, aggression, withdrawal or repeatedly asking for attention — are actually untreated pain. Pain may be the biggest cause of such symptoms — as well as of language breakdown. The problem is that not all health professionals or care partners are yet aware of this, so while pain may be the underlying cause of some behaviour, people with dementia might be given inappropriate sedating medication instead.

We know how to 'cure' Alzheimer's or some other dementia

There is no cure for dementia and currently no medicine that will reverse it. However, there are some medicines that may be used to help slow down some types of dementia. One care partner told us:

> *There were a large number of 'helpful' people who meant well but persisted in sending me all the latest fads they found on the internet which were going to cure him. Invariably, I had to very politely inform them that the 'cures' were at best suggestions for improving health in older people with mild cognitive impairment.*

To cure dementia all we need to do is spend more money on research

Of course everyone would like there to be a cure, but we also need more research on the non-pharmacological and positive, psychosocial interventions for dementia to improve wellbeing and quality of life, and not only research for a cure, but research for improving care.

Living beyond or well with dementia is not possible

Untrue. There are hundreds, in fact, more likely millions living with dementia, and living well and beyond their diagnosis. We'll discuss this topic more below.

Recently, many people living with dementia have been having global conversations with others diagnosed with dementia about the terms 'living well with dementia', or 'living better with dementia', these terms are not palatable for everyone with dementia, whereas 'living beyond dementia' seems to be more acceptable. If you have a diagnosis of dementia, we invite you to join these global conversations at www.joindai.org.

Sharing the diagnosis

When telling your family and friends you have dementia, there are a number of different reactions, but for those closest to you, they will also experience shock and anger, and as the disease progresses, anticipatory grief.

One daughter's reaction to hearing about her older mother's diagnosis: 'It was not a shock. But it was a painful truth.'

One man, diagnosed with younger onset dementia, aged 36 said:

> *I felt like throwing myself off a cliff…how the hell could someone my age have dementia?! It was a huge shock, and I am still coming to terms with it, though…some days I even forget I have dementia, those days it is not as bad as I first feared. BUT! The bad days are like, bloody shocking! I worry about my kids all the time, and about how my wife will cope, you know, later on.*

The responses from others vary. Some family and friends are over protective, immediately wanting to help, to take over for the person diagnosed, and try to somehow love them more. Some 'friends' start avoiding you, not through unkindness, but perhaps because of fear of what is ahead, a lack of awareness about dementia, or simply not knowing what to say.

The advice for anyone reading this book is to just say hello to the person diagnosed, as you would if they were diagnosed with any other terminal illness or chronic progressive disease, or at any other time you meet. It is now that people with dementia really need your friendship and support.

The late Dr Richard Taylor who was diagnosed with younger onset dementia always said, especially when someone said to him, 'I don't know what to say', 'Just say hello.' Most people actually just need company and support, and at some stage will want to talk about it.

Some people may openly accuse people with dementia of lying, or suggest the doctor is wrong. Many say, 'but I forget things too', or 'my mother/father/grandmother is like that'. If you remember something in a conversation, some will say, 'see, you can't possibly have dementia'. These responses are unhelpful, and to the person diagnosed, usually hurtful and insensitive.

With most other common diseases, almost nobody is diagnosed at a late stage. Unfortunately, some people with dementia don't get diagnosed until later in the disease, but as public awareness increases, and diagnostic processes improve this is changing. However, many people still have a stereotype of people with dementia that corresponds to more severe stages of the disease.

An older mother of an adult child who was diagnosed with younger onset dementia said she felt 'an anger and feeling of deep sadness like she had never felt before' when told her daughter had dementia. She still cannot imagine placing her daughter into aged care and has found the isolation and stigma has impacted her as the mother. She talked about the 'wall of silence' in the community she lives in, and no-one wanting to talk about her daughter any more. There are few, if any, supports for older parents of adults with younger onset dementia, and this group is facing their own ageing and health issues, on top of this grief.

The following are two reactions in the family of Kate Swaffer after she was diagnosed with younger onset dementia aged 49.

One son said, 'But Mum, isn't that a funny old person's disease?'

They had never realised younger people are also diagnosed with dementia and, even though Kate had worked in aged and dementia care previously, she had not realised it.

Kate's husband said some time later, 'I know I am losing you, and I am afraid of what the future holds.'

One mother with younger onset dementia very tearfully said; 'I had no idea I could get dementia…who is going to look after my small children?'

This young woman has three young children, all who were below the age of 13 when she was diagnosed two years ago and, although her husband still works, he now needs to work less to support her. The tears and sadness in her eyes were overwhelming and yet she was strong and determined to 'be their mum' for as long as possible.

One of the most helpful ways of coping with life for the person diagnosed with dementia or their family and supporters is to get support from others facing dementia, as well as from your family and friends.

That may mean being up-front about the diagnosis, and as one man (a friend of a person with dementia) said:

> *If we don't know anything is wrong, or that you are sick, or how bad it really is, or how you feel, how on earth can we support you?*

For the person diagnosed with a dementia, speaking and meeting with others with dementia to share your experience can be therapeutic and helpful. Dementia Alliance International[5] (DAI), an advocacy and support group, of, by and for people with dementia, hosts weekly online support groups and other events to specifically support people with dementia. They also now host online support groups for people with Primary Progressive Aphasia.

In this changing world of funding and policy, it is hugely beneficial for people with dementia to easily be able to get support that costs nothing and is easy to access if they have a computer and internet access. DAI also have private Facebook groups for people with dementia to join and share support.

One person with dementia, who was feeling like there was nothing left to live for said:

> *Meeting and speaking to others facing the same as me, in a confidential, relaxed, online group, in the privacy of my own home, felt like it saved my life. Knowing I didn't have to watch what I said, as we have all got dementia, makes it easier, and more helpful.*

Care partners also report that it is helpful to share the challenges and changes to their roles and life with others who are going through the same thing. There are various groups for families and care partners being run in Australia, many of them through Alzheimer's Australia[6], as well as many

---

5 *Dementia Alliance International http://www.joindai.org*

6 *Alzheimer's Australia https://fightdementia.org.au/services/carer-support-groups*

private Facebook and other online support groups for care partners and people with dementia. See the Resources section at the back of the book.

Prescribed Disengagement[7]®

There is a belief in the community, as well as in the health sector, that people with dementia cannot live positively with a diagnosis of dementia, and certainly not live well or beyond dementia with a truly productive and meaningful life. The diagnosis of dementia, and the Prescribed Disengagement that comes with it means that most people have been told and believe dementia is only a pathway to aged care and death. You may ask, what is Prescribed Disengagement?

When Kate Swaffer, one of the authors of this book, was first diagnosed, she was told to 'give up work, give up studying at the University of South Australia, to get her end of life affairs in order, and on the way, get acquainted with aged care'. Bear in mind, she was aged 49. At no time was she told it was a terminal illness, nor was she or her family given the appropriate support for it being one, even though it was repeatedly made very clear to them all she should 'get her end of life affairs in order' sooner rather than later. Her husband was also told he would very soon have to give up his work, and become a full time carer. Many individuals with dementia have reported this experience of being told to give up, and the care partner and other families report being advised to take over.

The cost of this Prescribed Disengagement is that it can cause a sense of hopelessness, and no hope of a future, and can readily mean the person diagnosed takes on the victim or sufferer role, and the care partner takes over control, and sometimes the martyr role. This is not only unhelpful, it disempowers and disables the person diagnosed, and gives all the power to the person without dementia. It prescribes that they take over, so care partners are simply doing what the 'system of support' tells them to do. The real cost of this is a sense of no hope or any sense of a good future, and for the person diagnosed, it also creates learned helplessness. If someone always corrects you, or takes over for you because it is easier and quicker

---

7 *Registered Trade Mark of Kate Swaffer*

for them, and they have been told they will have to, then many with dementia simply give up trying to help or speak for themselves, or to learn to live beyond dementia.

This Prescribed Disengagement has the potential to emotionally disable the person diagnosed, leading them to learned helplessness and to take on the sick role. Overmier defined learned helplessness like this:

> *Learned helplessness arises from experiencing unpredictable and uncontrollable events — usually traumatic ones — and is reflected in reduced ability to cope with future life challenges; these challenges could be behavioural, psychological/ cognitive, or health related. The demonstrations that experiencing uncontrollable, unpredictable traumatic events leads to future failures to cope with environmental challenges are of considerable importance empirically and theoretically and they inform psychological treatment of depression and post-traumatic stress disorder and psychological science.*

Prescribed Disengagement lowers a person's own expectations about how they can live. It lowers others' expectations about how they can function and live. This includes families and friends, employers, health-care professionals and service providers. It influences the services and support that people with dementia receive. For example, if you were still working and had experienced a stroke, you would have been authentically rehabilitated and supported to return to work, in whatever capacity possible, if that was your wish. Your employer would have been legally obliged to provide reasonable adjustments for you to continue to work, and to support any disAbilities. People with dementia are also less likely to be offered rehabilitation after hip surgery than people without dementia, even though they improve with rehabilitation.

If when they are diagnosed, people with dementia are told there is no hope, advised to give up their pre-diagnosis lives, and then only counselled to prepare for end-of-life and aged care, it is highly possible that many people diagnosed with dementia will develop learned helplessness. Family members then end up accidentally supporting

Prescribed Disengagement and supporting the learned helplessness, not because they mean to disable and disempower the person they love with dementia, but because they are advised they will have to take over, and so they do.

One woman with younger onset dementia said, 'Why is it that one day I was working full-time and raising my kids, and the next day told to go home and give up.' This is well meaning advice, but it is also illogical and extremely unhelpful.

Prescribed Disengagement supports and exacerbates ignorance, social inequality, exclusion, stigma, isolation, fear and discrimination. Dementia is the only disease Kate Swaffer knows of where you are actively and frequently told to *give up* rather than *fight for your life*.

One psychiatrist told us:

> *To be diagnosed with dementia is often associated with receiving a death sentence, people are told to get their lives in order and prepare, as if for the plague. This often translates — for the person given the diagnosis — as a sense almost of learned helplessness, a sense of 'losing oneself' and having your life taken over by others as you are considered to not have the full capacity for controlling your own destiny any longer.*

We need to break this negative and destructive cycle, and it has to start at the time of diagnosis; the immediate post-diagnostic support needs to reflect a more ethical pathway of support that is proactive, rehabilitative, enabling and that empowers the person with dementia and their families that it is possible to live beyond dementia in a more positive way, at least until the disease progresses too much. This type of support may even slow the progression down, and there is enough anecdotal and emerging evidence now to support this.

Alternative pathways of support may not be a cure, but they have huge potential to change the current trajectory of disempowerment, disablement and suffering on the way to death, to one that supports living more positively.

The following two graphics outline the current medical model of care, comparing it with a pathway of support designed by Kate Swaffer, based on social and disability support, to live with dementia, not only to die from it.[8]

Current medical model of 'care'

Diagnosis	
Often lengthy process of misdiagnosis	Most feared disease >65 age group

Assesments				
Driving	Medications	Activities of daily living	About dementia	Occupational therapy

Prescribed Disengagement®	
Not supported to live pre-diagnosis life	Lack of proactive or ethical pathway of care

Referral to service providers		
Alzheimer's Australia	Aged care provider	Community care provider

Advanced Care Directives

Aged care			
Community	Respite	Residential	Palliative care

8 *Adapted from K Swaffer,* What the Hell Happened to my Brain?: Living Beyond Dementia, *Jessica Kingsley Publsihers, UK, pp. 165–166*

Social/disAbility pathway of support

Diagnosis/confirmation of diagnosis

Access to UN CRPD	Access to disAbility support	Ethical pathway of support

Assessments

Driving	Medications	Activities of daily living	Information about dementia	Occupational therapy

Support for a terminal progressive chronic illness

Counselling for loss and grief and terminal illness	Assessment of disAbilities	Focus on quality of life	Support to remain employed if working	Support to stay engaged with pre-diagnosis lives

Rehabilitation

Speech pathology	Brain injury rehabilitation	Neuro-physio therapist	Neuroplasticity: new learning	Occupational therapy	Lifestyle changes: known risk reduction strategies

Strategies to manage and support disAbilities

Technology	Brain injury rehabilitiation	Electronic reminders	Walking stick	Buddy/ mentor	Webster packs	Support groups

Continued meaningfully engaging activities that give real value to living

Usual hobbies	Volunteering	Employment	Sport	Clubs	Usual socialising

Advanced Care Directives

Aged care

Community	Respite	Residential	Palliative care

An analogy used by others living with dementia or writing about dementia is of the swan, calm on top of the surface of the water, but paddling its feet furiously below the surface to stay afloat. Living with the symptoms of dementia can feel and look like that. People try and stay calm and unruffled and function smoothly, but as the symptoms progress, change or increase, the paddling underwater gets much harder. Paddling in order to function is also very tiring, a significant reason for fatigue as the day progresses.

Also using the swan analogy, if the person with dementia stops paddling hard, e.g. goes on a holiday, reduces exercise, and is 'wrapped in cotton wool' by others doing too much for them, the same thing that happens to the swan when it stops paddling appears to happen to people with dementia: they sink.

That is, the symptoms take over from the person's already impaired ability to function. Not working on non-pharmacological and positive psychosocial interventions also may make the disease or the symptoms of the dementia progress more quickly. Kate Swaffer and her husband have found repeatedly that when she has too much 'down time', her symptoms present themselves more strongly, and she has much more trouble functioning, speaking and remembering.

Is it possible to live a good life with dementia?

There are many people with dementia who are standing up and speaking out as advocates who demonstrate that there is still a good life to live even after a diagnosis of dementia. They have not accepted the Prescribed Disengagement and given up their pre-diagnosis lives, or they have entered into new and very productive lives as advocates with the lived experience of dementia, and we recommend to everyone who has been diagnosed with dementia, to re-invest in living your own life, as well as demanding the disability supports you rightfully deserve, for as long as possible.

Helga Rohra, a dynamic woman from Germany diagnosed with Lewy body dementia on her fifty-third birthday, and Chair of the European Dementia Working Group said: 'I don't want to be a victim of dementia, I want to be a victor of dementia.' She spoke at the Alzheimer's Disease International conference in Perth in 2014, and it was clear she is refusing to become a victim of dementia.

Ms J said, 'I am sick of people suddenly telling me what is best for me now! It's obviously time I spoke up for myself, like I used to before I got dementia.' This lady is a funny, feisty, 86-year-old, and has, 'reclaimed her life', saying she 'wanted her life back as everyone wanted to take it away after I was diagnosed', and she is proactively living as well as she can with dementia, and still living alone. She has a lot of supports in place now enabling her independence, including community care services.

Faith Riverstone, a woman diagnosed with dementia, and also the care partner for her mother, writes an insightful blog on her experience of living with dementia, and she wrote recently[9]:

> *It often happens when we try to speak up for ourselves, to say what we'd like for our care. Rather than listened to, we are often disrespected, challenged, and our message dismissed. This is done, most often, by people without the disease.*

When we talk about living well, or living beyond dementia, we are not talking about money or lifestyle, but about living beyond it and continuing to live the same life as your pre-diagnosis one for as long as possible. Sure, get your wills and other end-of-life issues sorted out (see Chapter 5) because dementia is a terminal illness and one where you will most likely lose capacity, but there is no need not to work hard to slow down the deterioration. And if you want to get onto your 'bucket list' straight away instead, that's absolutely okay too.

The media portray a public image of dementia where people's lives are devastated by the *suffering* of dementia, but there is so much more to life. In between the sadness and the deterioration caused by the symptoms, many people with dementia continue to live good and meaningful lives. As with any terminal disease or chronic illness, there are bad days, but they are not always like that.

---

9 *F Riverstone,* 'Ways In Which Others Dis-Able, and Dis-Empower, People With Dementia or Alzheimer's', *2015 https://stilllifewithdementia.wordpress.com/2015/12/05/*

Chapter 3

SUPPORT FOR LIVING WITH THE DISABILITIES OF DEMENTIA

Assessment and support of disAbilities

If the symptoms of dementia were treated as disAbilities, the negative impact on the person, their family, and society would be far less. People with dementia would be given assistance to remain employed, or fully engaged with their pre-diagnosis lives, if that is still their wish, which in turn would increase social inclusion and social equality. This would decrease the isolation, stigma, and discrimination, which in turn would decrease the economic impact on person and society.

People with dementia need strategies and support to assist them to live with the unique challenges of dementia, and this includes a disAbility plan, and may include assisted technologies, disAbility equipment, mentoring, and even recording conversations (for example with their doctor) to allow them more independence.

For example, the University of South Australia disAbility support services provided the following pathway for Kate Swaffer, which has enabled her to continue studying, and succeeding at university:

- referral to a disability adviser to provide support to continue with meaningful engagement (studying)

- mentor and buddy
- Disability Access Plan (diagnosis accepted with medical confirmation)
- alternative assessments and exams
- loss and grief counselling
- note taker and/or podcasts
- strategies for students, including, planning for completion of your degree, time management, managing reading and writing, study skills, library assistance, etc.
- supportive aids, as required
- disability equipment and assisted technology.

The immediate value of this proactive and enabling support is that she learned to see the symptoms of dementia simply as disAbilities, rather than just the pathway to aged care and death. It taught her how to manage them in order to continue functioning productively and meaningfully (to her), and doing something that was of real value to her. It also reduced stigma, discrimination, isolation and loneliness, significantly reduced the shame and social inequality she was feeling and the feeling that she was losing her identity. It allowed continued, meaningful positive engagement that had inherent value to her, and gave her a sense of achievement. Studying is also in line with the evidence that learning new things induces brain cell and connection growth, which may slow the progression of symptoms. There is no doubt it has helped her avoid apathy and depression.

The recognition of the symptoms as disAbilities would assist with a more equitable and dementia-friendly and dementia-enabling experience for the person with dementia after diagnosis. In contrast to the medical model, the disAbility pathway of support is positive and supports continued engagement and active meaningful living. This would ensure people with dementia are treated with dignity and as whole and individual human beings, people with the same disability rights as every other person with a disability.

Focus on QoL and wellbeing (for both the person with dementia and their care partner)

Doctors sometimes focus only on physical aspects of health, and on managing 'problems' and less on overall quality of life and wellbeing. We believe that it is really important for people with dementia and their care partners to focus on living a good life, so much so we have devoted the whole of Chapter 11 to this topic.

Support to remain employed if working

Please see the section on employment and dementia in Chapter 8.

Support to stay engaged in pre-diagnosis life

There are not yet any formal services to support you to stay engaged in your pre-diagnosis life, or to live beyond a diagnosis of dementia positively, so this is something that you will need to do with your informal social supports. Ignoring Prescribed Disengagement may be the first step towards this. First make a commitment to stay engaged in your pre-diagnosis life as much as possible, if, of course, that is what you want to do.

Some people will simply head for their bucket list when diagnosed with a terminal illness, or will respond and want to live differently. That's okay too, but, the message is, don't give up living your life, whatever that means to YOU personally. Then keep working on the right balance for you at each point in time between being active, and being so active and challenged that it is detrimental to your wellbeing.

Hopefully your care partner and family and friends will also read this book or, at least this chapter so that they understand why you might be trying so hard to stay active rather than taking the advice that is so commonly prescribed.

Speak with other people with dementia who are also working hard at staying active — so that in your social world it is 'normal' for people with dementia to be living well. Observe how they manage when things become difficult, and offer them your support as well. Join exercise groups or social clubs, as they will ensure you get out of the house, and will help with things like fitness and making new friends.

Rehabilitation for dementia

The World Health Organization (WHO) defines rehabilitation[10] as:

Rehabilitation of people with disabilities is a process aimed at enabling them to reach and maintain their optimal physical, sensory, intellectual, psychological and social functional levels. Rehabilitation provides disabled people with the tools they need to attain independence and self-determination.

Looking at this definition, it is clear not only that people with dementia would benefit from rehabilitation, they have a human right to it.

If a person has had a stroke, they will be rehabilitated optimally, and if younger, supported to go back to work, with reasonable adjustments that allow them to do so, if at all possible. Currently, people diagnosed with dementia are simply told to give up or 'slow down'. They have a human right to access the same disability rights, and disability discrimination legislation as any other person, and a right to recognition under the United Nations Conventions of the Rights of Persons with DisAbilities (CRPD). Globally there is a lot of advocacy and work towards changing this.

Since rehabilitation is not currently provided for most people with dementia, if you want to use rehabilitation services, you will have to find an allied health professional, either with expertise in dementia, or who is willing to learn how to help you. You may even have to educate the health providers and allied health professionals about dementia, and about the rehabilitation help that you want. In Australia the Medical Benefits Scheme (MBS) provides Medicare rebates for five allied health visits a year for patients with chronic and complex care needs whose GPs have a GP management plan and team care arrangements. It is unlikely that your GP will have experience in making referrals for dementia, so you will also have to educate your GP or specialist on the referrals to allied health professionals that may help you.

There are usually rehabilitation services available as a private patient,

---

10 *World Health Organization*, Health Topics: Rehabilitation, *2015 www.who. int/topics/rehabilitation/en*

although you may need a referral to them from your neurologist or other medical practitioner to access them through your private health care provider, to avoid paying full fees. Once Kate Swaffer's specialist came on board with her rehabilitative approach to living with dementia, he referred her to the Memorial Hospital Brain Rehabilitation unit in North Adelaide, which was for an intensive program for ten weeks, three–four times a week, plus two hydrotherapy sessions. This included assessment by the rehab physician in the unit, and cost very little out-of-pocket expenses other than transport to get there. Ask your doctor if you want information about this type of support in your area.

If you qualify for a consumer directed home care package, you can ask for these allied health services to be part of your package (see Chapter 9 on services). A senior manager in a residential aged care group described the services that their clients most need and want:

> *The audit related to our residential aged care facility residents presenting with hip fractures recommended, 'Patients admitted from residential aged care facilities should not be excluded from rehabilitation programs in the community or hospital, or as part of an early supported discharge program.'*

The manager talked about how important it is to consider rehabilitation in relationship to a resident's return to function following surgery, whether they have dementia or not, and that it will improve outcomes, mobility and wellbeing for residents if they return to full function after something like a hip fracture. Although access to allied health is limited in aged care, it is worth providing post operatively for a resident in a specialised rehab unit, as those who have undertaken rehabilitation will move more quickly back to the facility, and is worth continuing within the facility, if possible. We have detailed the various allied health and other health options below. Do use rehabilitative supports such as physiotherapy, hydrotherapy, pilates, balance and strength exercises, and cardio exercise such as walking or even running.

Regardless of what condition, illness, injury or health crisis you have, having access to rehabilitation to live the best life possible, with the support you need, will improve outcomes and wellbeing. It may not cure dementia, but rehabilitating the symptoms of dementia as disAbilities gives everyone the best chance of living a good life.

Speech pathology

'Our communication is what humanises us, and large portions of our brain are devoted to it', says Anne Kavanagh, a speech language pathologist in Cairns.

Speech pathologists are allied health professionals who work with people who have difficulty communicating effectively or who have difficulty with feeding and swallowing.

Speech is a complicated muscle activity; to say our words aloud we need to have a program of sound patterns stored within our brain to produce each sound we make (i.e. how and where to move our tongue, and our lips, to shape the breath vibrating through our vocal cords into sounds). Then we have to sequence all those sounds together into a word. Next we need to string together words into sentences, according to the grammar rules of our language, so that people around us can understand what we're trying to tell them. While all this is going on, inside our minds we are formulating the next idea to convey, and it all happens in milliseconds! When dementia hits there may come a time when any, or even all, of the brain functions that are involved in your ability to tell people what you are thinking, and understand what they are saying, will be affected.

One lady said, 'One of the things I hate the most about dementia, is not being able to find my words and make myself understood…people can't be bothered after a while.'

Speech pathologists can help people with dementia with their communication. The speech pathologist determines which parts of your communication skills are working well and which are not, and then prescribe some activities or strategies that could help you maintain, improve or manage within your abilities. For example, they may help you practice and 'relearn' words that have been lost, or prepare 'memory books' to help you remember important information.

Speech pathologists can work with a person who has swallowing difficulties to ensure safe swallowing. Speech pathologists can also train care partners to communicate more effectively with their person with dementia.

We strongly recommend that if you are having language or speech difficulties, including word finding, you seek support from a speech pathologist soon after diagnosis. It is in the early stages of the dementia you will have the best chance of learning new strategies to support yourself. Even if these issues do not overly trouble you yet, learning and developing strategies to support language and speech changes will be an important part of maintaining a higher quality of life with dementia.

Brain injury rehabilitation

Dementia can be thought of as an acquired brain injury (ABI), even though it is not classified as such. ABI refers to any damage to the brain that occurs after birth (with the exception of Foetal Alcohol Spectrum Disorder). ABI can be caused by an accident or trauma, by a stroke, a brain infection, by alcohol or other drugs or by diseases of the brain like Parkinson's disease.

Damage to the brain caused by some of these diseases also results in dementia, for example, many who have a stroke will go on to get vascular dementia, and in fact, stroke is the leading cause of acquired brain injury in Australia[11]. Strokes occur when the supply of blood to the brain is stopped by a clot or bleeding, and it often results in physical disability as well as changes in a person's thinking and emotions.

The Reconnect Transition Program[12] in South Australia, which is funded by the Motor Accident Commission, helps people adjust to life after an ABI, assisting them to successfully reintegrate and reconnect with their communities. It is offered, at no cost, to people who have an ABI as a result of a road trauma incident. It would be really helpful to people with dementia if they were offered a similar service.

11 Brain Injury Australia, About Acquired Brain Injury, 2015 www.bia.net.au
12 Brain Injury SA, Reconnect Transition Program, 2015 http://braininjurysa.org.au

Neurophysiotherapy

Neurological physiotherapists or Neurophysiotherapists are physiotherapists who have specialised in neurological disorder, i.e. they are experts in movement and function and who manage people with movement disorders as a result of injuries and diseases of the brain, the spinal cord and the broader neuromuscular system. Caring for people with dementia is emerging in this field of physiotherapy. Kate Swaffer's personal experience is that this form of therapy has been of significant value in supporting her to live beyond dementia.

Neurophysiotherapists are interested in supporting safe mobility for people with neurological conditions, and work as part of a clinical interdisciplinary rehabilitation team.

Neuro physiotherapists support and teach people how to maximise their recovery and or potential. They use the knowledge of neuroscience and brain plasticity to improve mobility, help people to learn new skills, to transition in their lives as much as possible and to engage in what is important to them — their personal goals and individual expectations. They support improving mobility in a way that enables you to be independent and safe, without falling over and causing injury, and to have the confidence to continue to remain active. Dr James McLoughlin, a clinical neurophysiotherapist and academic at Flinders University said:

> *Dementia has previously not been prescribed rehabilitation — which we need to reverse. Only 17 years ago, there were only five papers on rehab for multiple sclerosis whereas now there are about three new papers per day — this needs to happen for dementia. Improving and maintaining function is possible, and evidence is much clearer in supporting this, including for people with dementia, not just other neurological disorders.*

Neuroplasticity: training your brain through new learning

We used to think that the brain could not grow new brain cells (called neurons). We now know that as we age we keep growing new neurons as well as forming new connections between neurons, albeit at a slower rate than when we were younger. We call the brain's ability to grow and change neuroplasticity. Neuroplasticity happens in relation to new experiences i.e. the brain rewires itself as we learn.

We know that people with early dementia have neuroplasticity. This means that their brains continue to grow and change as they acquire new information, though this neuroplasticity may be less than for people without dementia (i.e. they learn less easily). Practice, practice, practice! It may take longer (more practice) to form the connections in your brain, but they can be formed. If you're trying to learn new information, link it to other information you already know, for instance, if you're learning a person's name, think of other people who have the same name and picture them together.

It is plausible that if people with dementia continue to expose themselves to new information, and try to keep learning, that they may be able to keep forming new cells and connections and to a small extent combat the brain loss that accompanies the disease. However, we don't yet have evidence that people with dementia who do more new learning progress slower than people who don't.

People often ask if doing crosswords or Sudoku can prevent dementia. Crosswords and Sudoku only exercise one part of your brain — just like flexing your ankle. It would be better for your brain to exercise lots of different parts of it by doing a range of new things, which are mentally and/or physically challenging. For instance, volunteering in a new role, or learning how to dance. Further, you may get more benefits in terms of growing new brain cells or connections if you do things that are new rather than familiar. So if you have never done Sudoku before, you will get more benefits from learning to do them than if you've been doing Sudoku every day.

So, there is some suggestion that people with dementia may benefit from continuing to do things that are mentally challenging. This could mean doing some study, or learning to use a new piece of technology or computer program. You may also want to try and relearn a skill which you've gotten rusty at (such as playing the piano). As adults we get used to being expert at things and doing things easily and forget how it feels to be a novice at something. You don't have to be 'good' at something to enjoy doing it, or get benefits from doing it.

You may be interested in reading the two books written on Neuroplasticity by Dr Norman Doidge (see resources) for other ideas for supporting yourself, or a person with dementia in this way.

Occupational therapy

Occupational therapists are allied health professionals who specialise in helping people function to their maximum ability in everyday life — this may mean helping them be able to work, take public transport, do everyday activities including housework, manage their appointments and their personal care.

The occupational therapy service most commonly offered to people with dementia is home safety. The occupational therapist does home visits and assesses for safety, most commonly risk of falls. The therapist then makes suggestions about ways to make the home safer; this may include stair rails, shower rails, shower chairs, raising or lowering the heights of beds, chairs and tables, removing trip hazards such as carpets or wires, and improving lighting. The occupational therapist may also train the person with dementia and their care partner on how to do things safely (e.g. get in and out of the shower).

Occupational therapists can also help people with dementia tailor strategies for their individual situation (for examples of these see Chapter 6), such as helping them rearrange and de-clutter their wardrobe to make dressing easier and making a laminated list with the order in which to get dressed. Occupational therapists are particularly good at figuring out which step in an activity a person with dementia may be having difficulty with (e.g. when making a cup of tea, the main problem may be remembering where everything is kept), and helping them overcome those difficulties (e.g. putting out the ingredients for the tea in the one spot on the kitchen bench). They call this task modification.

Occupational therapists may be able to conduct an assessment and prescribe meaningful activities that engage people with dementia (things that they can do that they enjoy). They may also be able to conduct assessments of behavioural and mood changes in dementia and try and figure out how to change the person's environment or use other psychosocial strategies to reduce these changes (see Chapter 4 on behaviour and non-pharmacological strategies for more on these). It would be even more helpful if a stronger focus were placed on living well with dementia and living independently.

Cognitive rehabilitation

Cognitive rehabilitation is usually delivered by psychologists or neuropsychologists. This involves identifying cognitive rehabilitation goals of the person with dementia, and then formulating and trialling strategies to help them achieve those goals. Usually interventions draw upon a mixture of approaches aimed at restoring lost function, using compensatory strategies and environmental modification to make the task easier. Errorless learning (see page 120 for more) and spaced retrieval techniques may be used. Problems that the person with dementia may want to work on may be related to their memory (e.g. I'm finding it hard to remember appointments), or problem solving (e.g. I find it difficult and stressful to make even small decisions like what to buy at the shop), or behaviour (I become really tired in the afternoon and find it hard to think or talk properly).

Lifestyle

An active lifestyle may help slow the progression of dementia. Perversely, Prescribed Disengagement may exacerbate the symptoms of dementia or result in faster decline.

There is a growing body of evidence suggesting that lifestyle factors are related to memory and thinking in older people, and to risk of dementia. There is also an emerging body of work suggesting that remaining physically and mentally active and eating a healthy diet will slow the decline in people with mild cognitive impairment or dementia.

While the evidence for all these factors is not strong yet, given that there is good evidence that (with the exception of cognitive training) these lifestyle changes improve our physical and/or mental health, we strongly recommend that people with dementia don't give up on these lifestyle factors.

Physical activity

Research suggests that exercise is associated with improved brain health and is beneficial for cognition in older people. The research also suggests that exercise slows cognitive decline in Alzheimer's disease, and may decrease falls, improve depression, and daily function. We don't know what type of exercise is best — aerobic exercise (exercise that gets your heart rate going) and resistance training (strength building such as lifting weight) and flexibility and balance exercises (such as stretching and yoga) may all have some benefits. There are also some studies suggesting that specific types of exercise practice such as Tai Chi or dance (it doesn't seem to matter what type of dance — folk, tango, ballroom) may have some benefits for people with dementia.

Interestingly, one form of exercise that research is finding very useful for people with dementia is walking and interval walking (very fast walking for five–ten minutes, with breaks of slow walking for 30–60 seconds). Walking should be encouraged in the early phases of dementia as not only will it help you keep or get fit, it has the potential to slow the symptoms of dementia. Even if you need someone to go with you so you don't get lost, we recommend you start walking.

We also don't know how often or for how long people with dementia should be exercising to get benefits, therefore suggest that as a minimum you try and meet general recommendations for physical activity.

Here are the Australian recommendations for physical activity for adults 18 to 64 years (even if you are over 64 years, you may like to try and meet these recommendations):

---

1. Doing any physical activity is better than doing none. If you currently do no physical activity, start by doing some, and gradually build up to the recommended amount.

---

2. Be active on most, preferably all, days every week.

---

3. Accumulate 150 to 300 minutes (2 ½ to 5 hours) of moderate intensity physical activity or 75 to 150 minutes (1 ¼ to 2 ½ hours) of vigorous intensity physical activity, or

---

an equivalent combination of both moderate and vigorous activities, each week. If you can comfortably talk, but not sing, you're doing moderate intensity activity. If you can't say more than a few words without gasping for breath, you're exercising at a vigorous intensity. Examples of moderate intensity physical activity are brisk walking, dancing, gardening, heavy housework. Examples of vigorous intensity physical activity are running, walking up hills, fast cycling, aerobics, fast swimming, competitive sports and games that require running (lawn bowls does not count!).

4. Do muscle strengthening activities on at least two days each week.

Here are the Australian recommendations for physical activity for Australians aged 65 and over:

1. Older people should do some form of physical activity, no matter what their age, weight, health problems or abilities.

2. Older people should be active every day in as many ways as possible, doing a range of physical activities that incorporate fitness, strength, balance and flexibility.

3. Older people should accumulate at least 30 minutes of moderate intensity physical activity on most, preferably all, days. (see above recommendations for what this means)

4. Older people who have stopped physical activity, or who are starting a new physical activity, should start at a level that is easily manageable and gradually build up the recommended amount, type and frequency of activity.

5. Older people who have enjoyed a lifetime of vigorous physical activity should carry on doing so in a manner suited

to their capability into later life, provided recommended safety procedures and guidelines are adhered to.

Simply put, exercise and physical activity are good for you, no matter how old you are, or whether you have dementia or not. In fact, staying active can help you:

- keep and improve your strength so you can stay independent
- have more energy to do the things you want to do
- improve your balance
- prevent or delay some diseases like heart disease, diabetes, and osteoporosis
- improve your mood and reduce depression.

You don't need to buy special clothes or belong to a gym to become more active. Physical activity can and should be part of your everyday life. Find things you like to do. Go for brisk walks. Ride a bike. Dance. Work around the house. Garden. Climb stairs. Swim. Rake the leaves.

Try different kinds of activities that keep you moving. Look for new ways to build physical activity into your daily routine. There are many resources to help people be physically active. Some other simple tips are to join a group, get a buddy, and use a pedometer or other device to monitor your levels of physical activity.

Cognitive training and cognitive stimulation therapy

We've already discussed the concept of neuroplasticity and why doing mentally challenging activities may be good for your brain above.

Cognitive training and cognitive stimulation are two specific ways of doing mentally challenging things.

Sometimes known as brain training, cognitive training provides structured practice on memory, attention and problem solving tasks. This is usually done on a computer, and the program can adjust the difficulty of the exercises based on the person's performance. Popular brain training programs include Lumosity and NeuroNation. However, please note that the claims that Lumosity can alleviate the symptoms of Alzheimer's disease have not been substantiated by research; see section on warnings in Chapter 4 for more details on this. There have been studies of cognitive training for people with dementia, and these show that doing memory exercises increase performance on memory tasks, doing attention exercises improves performance on attention tasks. However, these improvements on specific mental abilities do not generalise to general mental performance or how the person functions in everyday life. We don't know exactly what types of brain training exercises may have benefits, how often you need to do them, and for how long. There is a sensible rationale that brain training may help slow down the progression with dementia (the same rationale for which we suggested that you keep doing mentally challenging things) however we haven't got scientific proof this works.

Cognitive stimulation therapy is a program of group activities for people with dementia, which has been shown in several studies to improve cognition and quality of life of people with mild to moderate dementia. The social aspect of the program appears to be important, as the program has not been shown to be successful when presented by care partners to people with dementia individually. The program usually runs for two 90-minute sessions a week. There are a range of activities which engage memory, thinking and problem solving skills — for instance, developing a menu from a set of items based on a budget, or writing a story. There are not many services in Australia offering cognitive stimulation therapy, you could request that your local day care or other service set up a group — an experienced facilitator of groups of people with dementia could run the program, and detailed manuals are available. See http://www.cstdementia.com/page/the-manuals.

Social engagement

Social engagement means participating in social activities and having relationships with people where you do things in real life together. Older people who are more socially active (either because they have a larger social network, or because they socialise more often) tend to live longer, be more satisfied with life, have better cognition and have lower risk of dementia.

Many intervention studies for people with dementia (e.g. exercise or cognitive training) also increase social engagement, but no studies have examined the effect of purely increasing social engagement on how dementia progresses. We know that any social interaction (e.g. reading someone a newspaper or just making conversation) can reduce levels of agitated behaviour, as well as reduce feelings of loneliness and sadness.

Focusing on maintaining levels of social engagement may also improve the quality of life, particularly in the areas of relationships and meaning in life.

Diet

Some foods have been consistently associated with decreased risk of dementia such as unsaturated fatty acids, antioxidants, vitamin B and vitamin D. The Mediterranean diet, which involves eating primarily plant-based foods, such as fruits and vegetables, whole grains, legumes and nuts, eating fish and limiting red meat and using olive oil rather than butter has also been shown to be associated with decreased risk of dementia. Smoking and eating foods with higher amounts of aluminium seem to increase the risk of dementia. Some foods have been investigated but the evidence is mixed about whether they relate to dementia or not — these are fish, vegetables and fruits, and alcohol (where some studies suggest that a moderate intake may be beneficial).

We don't know how long people need to have these dietary patterns in order to change their risk of dementia. We also don't know whether people with dementia change their diet they can improve their symptoms or slow the progression.

However, we do know that eating a healthier diet will improve how you feel as well as improve your overall health.

Since we don't know what the optimal diet may be for people with dementia, it would seem to be sensible to eat a healthy balanced diet. The Australian dietary guidelines suggest that a healthy diet involves eating a wide variety of foods including larger amounts of vegetables, legumes/beans and grains, particularly whole grains, and high fibre cereals, and smaller amounts of fruit, dairy foods (milk, yoghurt, cheese, cream), and lean meats and fish, eggs, tofu, nuts and seeds. Use small amounts of oil and other fats, and only very occasionally eat foods with saturated fat, added salt, added sugars and alcohol. Drink plenty of water.

Combining lifestyle changes

There is some evidence in older people suggesting that physical activity, cognitive activity and social engagement can have a synergistic effect i.e. that the sum is greater than the parts in terms of their effects on maintaining the brain. This has not been confirmed for people with dementia, but it would make sense that the synergistic effect would also apply. So if you are active in different ways, this may have greater impact than just doing lots of one type of activity.

Strategies to manage and support disAbilities

Our advice in this book is to work hard to 'live with', not only 'die from' dementia, to manage the symptoms as disAbilities, including asking for disability support, like any other disabled person would be actively supported with, in order to continue to function well and independently for as long as possible. Do not allow yourself or the person with dementia you are supporting, to be wrapped up in cotton wool and give up.

Although it can be hard work finding support with non-pharmacological interventions and remaining positive and meaningfully engaged, and even though it may not be a cure, it does have the potential to greatly improve quality of life and wellbeing, as well as a person's perceived longevity. Importantly it gives people a sense of hope. Once you take away a person's hope, they have very little left.

See Chapter 6 for more detailed advice.

Continue meaningfully engaging activities that give real value to living

If you are a person with dementia (or a care partner) reading this, try to keep doing activities that are meaningful to you and that you really enjoy doing. Doing things that you enjoy isn't just filling in time or doing leisure activities. They aren't just things that are 'nice' to do in your spare time. Think of these as pleasurable therapy. In residential care, many activities are seen as therapeutic from a funding and accreditation perspective.

Meaningful activities are therapy because they:
- Provide mental, social and physical stimulation, which can slow decline or improve mental function in dementia.

- Are pleasurable (either in the doing, or in the achieving) — and part of having a good life is to have pleasure.
- Are a way to develop or maintain a relationship. When making conversation becomes more difficult, because you can't remember things or can't concentrate, you can still do things as a way of connecting and spending time together.
- Can help stave off boredom. When we are bored, we are disengaged and disinterested in the world. Bored children usually 'misbehave', so do bored adults.
- Can distract from situations, events or other things that are stressful or difficult, and which may result in behaviour changes.
- Help you maintain your self-identity. What we do every day defines how we see ourselves as people. Don't let your self-identity just be defined by dementia.

Living your life, in the same way you did before diagnosis is perhaps, the best intervention for dementia of all, if that is what you still want to do. Some people, after a diagnosis, will want to change their lifestyle. For example, as mentioned before, they may want to get on with their 'bucket list', or simply spend more time relaxing or with family. That's okay too. Interests may also change after dementia, so a person may no longer be interested in activities that they once enjoyed.

If you're unsure about what activities may be meaningful and engaging to you, here are some questions to help you (and your care partner) figure this out:
- » What things get you really excited or really excited you in the past (e.g. going to watch your favourite football team, sailboats, baking a cake)?
- » Is there something that you've always wanted to try (e.g. tango dancing, snorkelling, patchwork)?
- » Are there places that you have always wanted to go?
- » What groups do you enjoy or have you enjoyed being a part of (e.g. soccer team, P&C, choir)? If you can no longer belong to that group, can you join a similar group?

» Is there something you want to learn (e.g. Spanish, how to knit, something on the computer, go to university)?
» Is there something you did when you were younger that you have always wanted to go back to (e.g. playing the piano, writing poetry, shortwave radio)?
» What would be an ideal day for you (e.g. I would wake up early, walk on the beach, have lunch with friends, do some gardening, have a quick game of tennis, study, go to work, volunteer, have dinner with family or friends, and then fall asleep?
» What would you like more of in your life (e.g. cuddles, laughs, quiet time)?

You may need to develop some life enhancement strategies to help you be able to continue with these activities. If it is a group activity, it may also help to talk to the people in your group so that they can help support your disAbility. We have heard many stories of bridge companions, golf buddies, men's sheds and craft groups supporting people with dementia to keep doing the activity as part of the group. Unfortunately, we have also heard stories of people with dementia who have been excluded because of their abilities. For instance, a lady who had sung in a choir for years was told she was not welcome in the group because she could no longer sing from memory and wanted to use a songsheet, and a gentleman who had played golf all his life but could no longer manage the score card, even though he had organised a friend to support him by scoring.

It is important to continue to spend time nurturing friendships and relationships, especially with those you love. Strategies to remain positive can be enhanced by building on your own resilience, as well as looking after your health and having time out from dementia.

Chapter 4

TREATMENTS AND PROGNOSIS

There is currently no cure for any common form of dementia. For some forms, there are treatments that may delay the progression of the condition.

Alzheimer's disease and mixed Alzheimer's disease and vascular dementia

There are four medications currently available for the treatment of Alzheimer's or Alzheimer's disease mixed with vascular dementia. Three of these drugs, Aricept, Exelon, and Reminyl, work in the same way, and are classed as acetylcholinesterase inhibitors, the fourth, Ebixa works slightly differently. There is also a product combining Aricept and Memantine called Namzaric, which is used for people with moderate-to-severe dementia. At the time of writing, Namzaric has not been approved for use in in Australia by the Therapeutic Goods Administration.

Acetylcholinesterase inhibitors

Acetylcholinesterase inhibitors act by increasing the amount of a neurotransmitter (chemical in the brain) called acetylcholine which is relatively low in people who have Alzheimer's disease. Acetylcholine is involved in memory functioning. The three acetylcholinesterase inhibitors approved for use by the therapeutic goods administration (TGS) in Australia are Aricept (generic name donepezil), Exelon (generic name rivastagmine) and Reminyl (generic name galantamine).

Acetylcholinesterase inhibitors compensate for a deficiency of one neurotransmitter, but do not change brain structure, or halt the cause of the brain deterioration. Hence acetylcholinesterase inhibitors only work for a period of about twelve months and then their effects wear off, probably because the brain continues to deteriorate. Areas that may improve with these medications include memory and thinking, and improved ability to initiate and be interested in things such as household chores or hobbies. Some people also experience small improvements in behavioural symptoms and their ability to conduct more complex activities of daily life (such as paying bills and cooking).

Acetylcholinesterase inhibitors don't seem to work for everyone with Alzheimer's disease. About a third of people with the condition improve for a period, one third stabilise, and one third don't seem to respond. We don't have a way of predicting who will benefit.

Side effects that can occur in a small percentage of people are lethargy, nausea, diarrhoea, vomiting, muscle cramps, dizziness, loss of appetite, insomnia and nightmares. These side effects are usually temporary and go away with time. About a third of people in clinical trials of the medications drop out because of side effects. People respond differently to the three acetylcholinerase inhibitors and may find fewer side-effects or greater clinical benefits from one or another.

Acetylcholinesterase inhibitors are subsidised by the Pharmaceutical Benefits Scheme (PBS) for patients with mild to moderate Alzheimer's disease. Six months of subsidised medication is approved initially. It is necessary for the prescribing doctor to judge that the medication has a clinical benefit to obtain continuation of subsidised treatment every six months thereafter. If you do not meet the criteria for subsidy, you can choose to pay for the drugs at full cost. Brand-name acetylcholinesterase inhibitors cost between one and five Australian dollars a pill depending on the brand, dose and quantity being bought.

Glutaminergic N-methyl-D-aspartate (NMDA) receptor antagonists

Glutaminergic N-methyl-D-aspartate (NMDA) receptor antagonists act by reducing the toxic actions in the brain of neurotransmitter called glutamate. Glutamate levels are relatively high in people who have Alzheimer's disease. The only glutaminergic N-methyl-D-aspartate receptor anatagonis approved for use by the therapeutic goods administration (TGA) in Australia is Ebixa (generic name memantine). Ebixa does not change brain structure or impact on the case of brain deterioration.

Ebixa has been shown to improve the memory and thinking, behaviour and ability to perform daily living tasks for people with moderate-to-severe Alzheimer's disease. Ebixa does not seem to have benefits for people with mild Alzheimer's disease.

Ebixa can be taken safely in combination with acetylcholinesterase inhibitors. The combination appears to provide synergistic benefits compared with the acetylcholinesterase inhibitor alone for people with moderate to severe Alzheimer's disease.

Other drug therapies

Many other drugs have been tested as potential treatments for Alzheimer's disease and there has been data from observational studies and laboratory studies supporting their potential effectiveness. These drugs include vitamin E, selegiline, nonsteroidal anti-inflammatory drugs, statin drugs, omega-3 fatty acids, hormone replacement therapy (HRT — estrogen or combined estrogen plus progestin therapy), and B vitamins. However, clinical trials have found little benefit, so their use is not recommended for dementia.

Complementary and alternative therapies

There are many complementary and alternative medicines that have been tested and/or promoted as having benefits for patients with Alzheimer's disease. Please be aware that vitamins and dietary supplements that you can buy off the shelf in a pharmacy do not require the same level of rigorous scientific research to support their claims of safety or effectiveness as prescription drugs. Their contents are also not as stringently regulated as prescription drugs.

Souvenaid is a nutritional drink that contains high levels of omega-3 polyunsaturated fatty acids, uridine monophosphate and choline, together with phospholipids, B vitamins and other nutrients. However, it may improve memory in people with mild Alzheimer's disease in those who have not previously taken cholinesterase inhibitors. It does not appear to have any benefits for people with moderate dementia. There is no evidence that it impacts on cognition more generally or daily function.

Side effects may be diarrhoea, constipation, flatulence, nausea, anxiety, depression, insomnia, hyperglycemia and weight gain. Souvenaid is not available on prescription and can be purchased over the counter from pharmacies or online. There is no government subsidy for Souvenaid, which currently costs about $4 a drink.

There is some evidence that Ginkgo biloba (a Chinese herb) helps reduce behavioural symptoms in people with dementia.

Alternative therapies which have been tested for Alzheimer's disease include, Huperzine A (derived from Chinese club moss) Brahmi (an Indian Ayurvedic herb), Choto-san and Kami-Umtan (both Japanese herbal preparations), acetyl-L-carnitine (a supplement), curcumin (derived from the turmeric spice), and coconut oil. Some of these medicines have been studied scientifically and have produced promising evidence from laboratory and animal studies. However, clinical trials in people with dementia have either not been conducted, negative or produced inconsistent results. So there is currently no convincing evidence for their use in humans.

Many people with dementia choose to take alternative or herbal therapies because they believe that they work for them, or 'in case' they may work. If you are considering taking these, please discuss this with your doctor, in case they interact with your existing medications.

Vascular dementia

The main aim of treatment for vascular dementia is to treat the underlying cause of the vascular changes to the brain, which means treating cardiovascular disease and managing cardiovascular risk factors such as high blood pressure, high cholesterol, smoking, being overweight, diabetes and lack of physical exercise. Treating cardiovascular disease and reducing risks can slow down the progression of vascular dementia, for instance by reducing the risk of future strokes or transient ischemic attacks (TIAs).

Most research into drug treatments for dementia has been focused on Alzheimer's disease with much less drug development and testing for vascular dementia. Acetylcholinesterase inhibitors and memantine produce small benefits in cognition of uncertain clinical significance in patients with mild to moderate vascular dementia and are not recommended treatments. Alternative treatments such as Chinese herbal medicines, Huperzine A and acetyl-L-carnitine have also been trialled for vascular dementia, but there is little evidence for their effectiveness.

Frontotemporal dementia

Since frontotemporal dementia is relatively rare, there has been relatively little research into developing new drug compounds specifically for the treatment of this form of dementia.

Drugs developed for Alzheimer's disease (acetylcholinesterase inhibitors and memantine) have been tested to see if they have benefits for people with frontotemporal dementia. The results suggest that they don't have any benefit.

Lewy body dementia

There is increasing research evidence suggesting that acetylcholinesterase inhibitors (donepezil, rivastigmine and galantamine — see the section on Alzheimer's disease, above, for more details) can help the attention and thinking of people with Lewy body dementia. These medications also seem to have some impact on decreasing hallucinations and agitation (behaviour changes in dementia will be discussed in greater detail below). However, people with Lewy body dementia may be at high risk of common gastrointestinal side effects of these medications such as nausea, vomiting, diarrhoea, anorexia and weight loss. They may also experience other side effects such as slow heart rate and other changes to the way the heart beats. Acetylcholinesterase inhibitors are not subsidised on the pharmaceutical benefits scheme in Australia for Lewy body dementia so people with this form of dementia will have to pay the full costs of these medications.

Memantine has also been trialled for Lewy body dementia, but any benefits are still uncertain.

Medications used for Parkinson's disease, such as carbidopa-levodopa (Sinemet) are used to treat movement symptoms in Lewy body dementia such as rigid muscles and slow movement, however they are usually less effective than in Parkinson's disease. People with Lewy body dementia and confusion, hallucinations and delusions may find these symptoms exacerbated.

Mood and behavioural changes in dementia

Mood and behavioural changes are very common in dementia, with estimates of these occurring in 90% or more people with dementia. It is important to acknowledge here, these mood and behavioural changes may not be due to the dementia or disease process, but rather a response to the way a person is being cared for, or how they feel about what is happening to them. For example, being forced to live in residential care facility may make a person angry and volatile. Many also suggest these changes are also due to communication breakdowns, and that the people supporting the person with dementia have not learnt to communicate with them in new ways.

Mood changes include being emotionally unstable, anxiety, sadness, and depression and, on rare occasions, elation. Behavioural changes include saying or doing things that are unsafe or not deemed socially appropriate, being verbally or physically aggressive, changes to sleep or eating patterns, seeing, hearing or feeling things that are not there (hallucinations), believing things are real that are not (delusions), restlessness and not being able to sit still and relax. These are collectively referred to as Behavioural and Psychological Symptoms of Dementia (or BPSD) and sometimes derogatively labelled 'challenging behaviours'.

The phrase BPSD appears to have been developed by pharmaceutical companies and clinicians, to draw attention to the behavioural changes which were then less recognised as occurring as a consequence of dementia, and to define people with dementia in ways that can be managed by drug therapies, for example using antidepressants or antipsychotics.

People with dementia often feel that being labelled with BPSD is disparaging, as they may feel that the way they have reacted or responded to something or someone, is due to their distress at what is happening, and not a symptom of the dementia at all. The label is more commonly used in residential aged care than when the person is living at home. Being ignored, forced to eat food you dislike, talked over or down to, or even made to engage in activities you find worse than boring and not to your own individual likes, may make some people angry, apathetic, or appear disengaged or non-compliant. In fact, it is often a normal response to what is happening, and the situation needs to change, not the person being labelled and managed. Better, more individualised care, that is more person- and relationship-centred would alleviate many of the so-called behaviours. Many people living in residential care spend hours doing very little other than sitting and waiting, and feeling bored and ignored; if we treated our children this way, they would 'misbehave' as well.

One man living in residential care who is still very functional said, 'Of course I'm gonna get stroppy with them, they make me get out of bed too early. I never got out of bed before around 11 before, so why would I want to start now just to suit them?!' Then he added, 'and I'm the one with dementia!'

The use of the term Behavioural and Psychological Symptoms of Dementia (BPSD) and labelling of behaviours such as wandering, aggression and screaming implies that the behaviours occur as an inevitable result of the disease, rather than partly because of the interactions of the person with dementia with the people around them and their environment. The labels can be disrespectful and also cause the person with dementia to be seen as a condition, e.g. a 'wanderer' or 'screamer', and decreases the likelihood of person-centred care being delivered. They also place the 'fault' of the behavioural changes on the person with dementia.

There is a growing a group of clinicians and researchers from around the globe who are also speaking up against the notion of BPSD, and believe that perhaps as few as 10% of people with dementia have challenging or severe behaviours due to the disease, and the other so called 'challenging behaviours' or BPSD are due to poor care, unmet needs including issues such as pain, or because those supporting people with dementia have not learnt to communicate with people with changed cognition.

Reasons for mood and behavioural changes

Mood (e.g. anxiety, sadness, depression) and expressions of distress can lead to behavioural changes for several reasons:

1. In reaction to the diagnosis of dementia, decline and difficulties with memory and thinking, and ability to function in the world e.g. a person with dementia may feel embarrassed because of his or her poor memory in social situations, and become anxious when having to interact with other people, or even in anticipating having to interact with others.

2. Changes to the brain structure or neurotransmitters e.g. serotonin neurons seem to be selectively lost in frontotemporal dementia. Serotonin is a neurotransmitter implicated in depression, though we still don't know the role it plays in the disease, or why selective serotonin reuptake inhibitors (SSRI) have improved depression symptoms.

3. Because the person is less able to cope with their environment, including the people in it e.g. in busy noisy environments such as a party, the person may have difficulty following one conversation or reading social cues while blocking out irrelevant information, so the person inadvertently says or does something which is not appropriate to the conversation.

4. Due to acute medical problems such as urinary tract infection, pneumonia, dehydration or constipation.

5. Due to unmet needs or distress, which the person may or may not recognise in themselves or cannot express such as discomfort, pain, hunger, fear, loneliness, boredom, need to go to the bathroom. A person with dementia may be unintentionally doing something really annoying to their care partner or the staff over and over because they are bored but don't recognise that they are bored or don't have the initiative to figure out

another way of occupying themselves. This may also be because there are no suitably interesting activities for the person to engage with. Being made to sit all day, or play bingo if you dislike bingo, for anyone, is annoying and boring.

6. Due to others (professionals, care partners, the community) not understanding what the person with dementia's needs or wishes are.

7. Due to others not understanding the person with dementia or knowing how to communicate with them; it is up to others to learn how to communicate with people with dementia, not the other way round.

8. Due to the lack of loss and grief counselling. We know that if new grief, or old unresolved grief is not treated or managed, it can cause symptoms similar to those of dementia, including apathy, depression, anxiety, sadness. If this grief goes untreated, then the symptoms of dementia may appear to be much worse than they actually are.

There may be many factors contributing to one's mood or behavioural symptom. For example, someone is afraid about what may happen in the future after he is diagnosed, and this makes him sad, fearful and depressed. Brain changes result in him having reduced initiative which means that he stops exercising which adds to his low mood or apparent apathy (as he misses out on endorphins and other benefits of physical exercise for mood). His spouse or the paid carer is hyper vigilant about 'watching' him to keep him safe, which undermines his self-confidence and exacerbates his fears and depression.

This is why we recommend that if you have dementia you seek support and counselling for the grief and loss, and the other changes caused by the symptoms of dementia, and you look after your emotional, psychological and physical health, as these may reduce or minimise mood and behavioural changes.

Behavioural or mood changes may also be more prominent at particular times of day, such as when the person is tired or feeling like there is nothing left in the tank.

Non-pharmacological (non-drug) strategies

Most dementia guidelines recommend that non-pharmacological strategies are trialled for managing mood and behaviour changes in dementia before drug therapy unless there is an urgent risk of harm to self or others, in which case drug treatments should be considered. However, many of our interviewees reported that more often drugs are introduced before non drug therapies are even considered. Please go to Chapter 6 where we discuss non-pharmacological strategies.

Pharmacological management of mood and behaviour

Drugs are commonly used as a management strategy for behavioural changes in dementia without trying non-pharmacological approaches first. This means that many people with dementia are taking medications, which they may not have needed to take, with concomitant risks of side effects.

Antidepressants for depression and other changes in dementia

Antidepressants have been shown to have limited benefit in the treatment of depression in dementia. Early studies suggested that selective serotonin reuptake inhibitors (SSRIs) did have an impact on depression in dementia, however recent research suggests that benefits may be minimal.

Antidepressants are sometimes also used to treat apathy and agitation in dementia but there is not much evidence that this is effective.

The side effects of Selective Serotonin Reuptake inhibitors (SSRIs) include nausea, dry mouth, insomnia, sleepiness or drowsiness, agitation, diarrhoea, excessive sweating and sexual dysfunction. SSRIs tend to be preferentially prescribed in older people because they are relatively safe for older people. Tricyclic antidepressants can worsen symptoms of dementia. Other side effects include postural hypotension (low blood pressure when standing) leading to falls and fractures, cardiac conduction abnormalities and delirium, urinary retention, dry mouth and constipation.

Antipsychotics for behaviour changes in dementia

Antipsychotics were originally developed for the treatment of schizophrenia. Of the many types of antipsychotic available, aripiprazole (brand name Abify) and risperidone (brand name Risperdal) have been shown to have small improvements on mood and behavioural symptoms with most of the evidence being for people with moderate to severe dementia. Only Risperidone is listed on the pharmaceutical benefits scheme as being subsidised for the treatment of behaviours in dementia.

There is also a black box warning for the use of antipsychotics for people with dementia. Antipsychotics are associated with a 1.7-fold increase in mortality compared to placebo and should only be used when absolutely necessary. Side effects associated with these antipsychotics including weight gain, diabetes and pre-diabetes condition, physical symptoms including tremor, slurred speech, muscle contractions which may result in pain, twisting, repetitive movements or abnormal postures, involuntary movements (including those of the face and jaw), restlessness, abnormal gait, stroke, and cardiovascular events.

People with Lewy body dementia have higher risks of side effects and have worse side effects from antipsychotic medication. People with frontotemporal dementia are also particularly susceptible to some of the side effects.

Despite warnings about side effects, about one third of Australian nursing home residents are regularly prescribed antipsychotics — this high rate is similar to the rate in other developed countries. Antipsychotics are commonly used by aged care staff to manage behaviours, sometimes before non-drug strategies are tried; this is a form of restraint, and if it is happening to someone with dementia that you support, then you should be asking questions, especially if it is prolonged use.

A care partner describes how not long after placing his wife into a nursing home, he was contacted by nursing home staff:

My wife was agitated and they wanted to give her some medication for that. So I said okay. They kept saying she was making too much noise, and that they give her this medicine to quiet her down. But they just kept giving her more and more and I noticed when I used to go see her, she'd just kind of mumble, like she was lost.

US Federal law prohibits the use of antipsychotics and other psychoactive drugs for the convenience of staff. It's called a 'chemical restraint.' There has to be a documented medical need for the drugs.

Australian law requires that written consent be obtained from a person responsible in order for an antipsychotic (or any other mind altering drug such as an antidepressant) to be prescribed to someone who can no longer consent for themselves. This written consent is usually not obtained in nursing homes. Many interviewees reported consent was never requested for the use of these drugs on a family member in residential care, and did not realise such actions are reportable.

Polypharmacy — taking more than one medication

People with dementia take, on average, one more medication compared to people without dementia of a similar age and taking into account physical health. There is also a high prevalence of inappropriate medication use in people with dementia. A medication is inappropriate where the harm of its use outweighs the benefit to the individual, or when a safer alternative exists. Often as people age their physical and cognitive functions change and medications that were once appropriate may become inappropriate.

Between 20 and 50% of people in the community with dementia, and over half of people with dementia in Australian nursing homes, take at least one inappropriate medication. The more medications you take (this is called polypharmacy), the more likely it is that there may be a negative interaction between two medicines. If different doctors prescribe your medicines (e.g. your GP, different specialists, a doctor at the hospital) they may not be considering all the interactions with other medicines.

If you have any concerns about the number or side effects of your medications, ask your GP to review all your medications to see if you continue to need them all. You can also ask for a home medicines review, which will involve you, your general practitioner and an accredited pharmacist and regular community pharmacy. The pharmacist's review and report is currently paid for by the Australian government.

Avoid medications with anticholinergic effects

There are some common medications that can make the symptoms of dementia worse. You may remember that earlier in this chapter we noted that medications for treating Alzheimer's disease increase the amount of the neurotransmitter acetylcholine in the brain. Some medications have anticholinergic effects, that is, they block the action of acetylcholine in the brain. This may make the symptoms of dementia worse. Some research suggests that about half of all people with dementia receive medications with anticholinergic effects.

Some examples of medications with anticholinergic drugs include:
- Benadryl (generic name diphenhydramine), an antihistamine used to treat allergies
- Xanax (generic name alprazolam), a benzodiazepine used to treat anxiety and panic disorders
- Congentin (generic name genztropine mesylate), used for treating Parkinson's disease
- Endep (generic name amitriptyline), a tricyclic antidepressant.

Miracle cures and scams

You will see all sorts of advertisements for miracle drugs these days; supplements that claim to stop or reverse ageing or dementia. You might even see statements like, 'This treatment cured XXX in one week.' Adverts like these appear to offer hope, but they are almost always false. Thanks (or not) to the internet, there are more ways than ever to sell untested products — online, TV, radio, magazines, and newspapers are just a few examples, and search engines allow scammers to prey on certain groups. Actors are even used to portray doctors and patients on infomercials. You might even get an email or a Facebook post urging you to try a product, and it is difficult to tell what's an ad.

Health scams set their sights on people who are scared, afraid, or in pain, and it's easy to see why a person with dementia might be tempted to believe in the promise of a miracle remedy. Health scams usually target diseases that may have treatments for symptoms but currently have no cure.

Untested remedies are usually also expensive, and very often a waste of money. They may be harmful, or get in the way of helpful drugs prescribed by your doctor. Occasionally a placebo effect will occur which will help with the symptoms. Please be careful, as dementia is the new 'disease with no cure' and there is most definitely big money in dementia.

Lumosity is one example of an intervention falsely claiming to have been shown to delay age-related cognitive decline and protect against mild cognitive impairment, dementia, and Alzheimer's disease. Lumosity is a computerised brain-training program endorsed in advertisements by Nicole Kidman and other celebrities. While there is evidence that some brain training programs can improve cognition in older people, there is no evidence that they delay decline or protect against dementia. The US Federal Trade Commission charged Lumosity with making unfounded claims, and Lumosity agreed to compensate consumers to the value of US$2 million.

Coconut oil is another intervention for which there are unsubstantiated claims that it benefits dementia or Alzheimer's disease. There are many scientific-looking articles online that report doctors talking up benefits of coconut oil. We identified one, small research study supporting this claim published in Tagalog in a Philippine journal. Coconut oil is about 90% saturated fat, and some research has suggested saturated fat increases risk of mortality, cardiovascular disease, coronary heart disease, stroke and type 2 diabetes. While the association between saturated fats and poor health is still being disputed, it would make sense to not take coconut oil as a treatment for dementia until its benefits and safety are rigorously demonstrated.

However, if you want to try any of these things, have the money for them, have checked they won't harm you in any way, and just want to give it a go, that is your choice. Many people swear by the benefits of some of these things, including simply enjoying doing them, or liking the taste of something like coconut oil in their cooking.

Here are some tips to protect yourself from health scams

Always be sceptical. Question what you see or hear anywhere, including newspapers, magazines, movies, radio and TV stations, as they do not always check to make sure the claims in their ads are true, nor do they say if a celebrity has been paid to endorse a product. Ask your doctor, nurse, other healthcare provider or pharmacist about a product before you buy it.

You may be supporting someone with dementia who is still living at home and gets caught by scams, and this can be a very difficult situation if they are still deemed to have legal capacity. This is a common situation and finding ways to support people that allow some protection from phone or internet scams may be worthwhile.

Don't let a salesperson or an ad talk you into anything, do your research and look for ads or promotional material that:

- claim to cure or even reverse any disease (such as arthritis or dementia) that hasn't been cured by medical science — we know there is currently no cure for dementia
- claim the product is made from a special, secret, or ancient formula
- offer products and services only by mail or from one company
- use statements or unproven case histories from so-called satisfied patients — always check their 'facts' and 'claims'
- promise you a no-risk, money-back guarantee
- offer an additional free gift or a larger amount of the product as a special promotion
- require advance payment
- claim there is a limited supply of the product.

If you have questions about a product, talk to your doctor or get advice from someone you trust. Getting the facts about healthcare products can help protect you from health scams, and save you a lot of false hope and money.

The Australian government has an agency that provides information about scams and works to protect consumers against them. You can also report a scam on their website: www.scamwatch.gov.au. The US Food and Drug Administration website also has information on health scams and lists 'medical' products and supplements that make misleading claims: http://www.fda.gov/ForConsumers/ProtectYourself/HealthFraud/.

Prognosis

Some of you reading this book will want to know what to expect. Others will not want to know or are not ready to think about this. We respect these choices, and suggest that those who don't want to know go straight to the next chapter.

Almost all dementias are a progressive, chronic and terminal disease. Decline can be gradual and insidious, or stepwise — with no changes for a while and then sudden deterioration. Sometimes changes happen quickly in a short period of time and then the symptoms plateau for a while. People with dementia also have good days and bad days, just like everyone else.

Here is how medical professionals view symptoms (disAbilities) by stage of dementia. These are broad descriptions, and people with dementia often progress differently to the stages described below:

Mild dementia

People with mild dementia have difficulty with their memory and thinking that interferers with more complex daily activities. For instance, completing the accounts, travelling or higher order work may be challenging, and require much more time or planning and support.

Moderate dementia

People with moderate dementia have trouble learning new things, and/ or remembering recent events. Their thinking ability is less complex and logical and their ability to remember the names of things or people may initially be what is most impaired. They may have trouble with self-care such as choosing the right clothes, or putting clothes on in the correct order. Their reduced judgement may mean that they need supervision to keep them safe. They may also not know the day or date, or where they are (if in an unfamiliar place).

Severe dementia

People with severe dementia cannot function without help. They have extreme memory difficulties and trouble expressing themselves and understanding others. The brain deterioration may have affected their motor control so the way they walk and move is affected, as is their ability to control their bladder and bowels.

End stage dementia

People with end stage dementia are bed bound. They may have trouble moving or controlling their limbs. They may no longer respond much to the outside world, both because their senses have dulled and deteriorated, and because they can no longer focus on things outside themselves. They will rarely try to communicate with or connect with other people. They may have trouble eating and swallowing and may refuse food or drink. Their whole body is breaking down and their breathing may become laboured. They may have pressure ulcers or bed sores. People with end stage dementia need everything to be done for them.

Palliative care during end stage dementia

The World Health Organization[13] defines palliative care like this:

> *Palliative care is an approach that improves the quality of life of patients (adults and children) and their families who are facing problems associated with life-threatening illness. It prevents and relieves suffering through the early identification, correct assessment and treatment of pain and other problems, whether physical, psychosocial or spiritual.*

During end stage dementia, care priorities should be making the person as comfortable as possible and pain free. Try and meet the person's emotional needs — let her know that she has people around her that love her. Use gentle touch, music and speech to try and connect, however briefly, with her.

---

13 *http://www.who.int/mediacentre/factsheets/fs402/en*

Decisions will need to be made about whether to undertake treatments that may prolong the person's life. See Chapter 5 on advance care directives and how the person with dementia can make these decisions for herself while cognitively able.

Decisions that may need to be made include:

» Whether to tube feed or not if the person can no longer eat or drink on her own. Tube feeding is not recommended for people with end stage dementia, as it does not appear to prolong life or improve other outcomes, and discomfort and other risks are associated with tube feeding. However, it can be heartbreaking for families to think that the person is going 'hungry'; hand feeding can be offered as an alternative

» Whether or not to use intravenous antibiotics. See section on pneumonia below for more information.

» Whether to resuscitate if the person stops breathing.

Most palliative care services operate from a health service, and many people with terminal illnesses choose to die in a hospice. For people with dementia, who may either be living at home or in residential care, this may not be the right choice. Having to cope with unfamiliar and new surroundings, new staff, new environments, and even simple changes like medical smells can be upsetting or confusing. Most people, if given a choice, say they would prefer to die at home (or on the golf course).

Most palliative care services will visit and support a person to die at home. Most residential care facilities also welcome external palliative care providers to attend to a dying resident. Ask your service provider, or contact the Palliative Care Association or services in your state about this.

People with dementia can live well at every stage, if you judge 'living well' according to the person's mood and comfort and, importantly, not according to the life they would have lived had they not developed dementia. This is true for those entering the last stage of their life, whether because of dementia, some other illness, or because of old age.

Alzheimer's Australia has a helpsheet, 'Caring For Someone With

Dementia 21: Palliative Care'[14] that you may find helpful. It provides some information on the palliative care approaches that play a crucial role in the care of the person who is dying, and provides information about how the person with dementia can be supported to die in comfort and with dignity.

How long do I have?

Studies of survival time for dementia have been from point of diagnosis. Average survival times in different studies have ranged from 1.1 to 8.5 years and in research studies the range of survival times ranges from 0.2 years to 11 years — though, anecdotally, we have heard of people living with dementia for more than 20 years.

Survival time cannot be predicted accurately. However, the severity of dementia at diagnosis, age at diagnosis, and type of dementia all seem to impact on survival time. Many die from something other than dementia, such as cancer or heart disease. Survival time does not appear to differ between men and women. The more severe the dementia at diagnosis, and the older the person at diagnosis, the shorter the survival period.

Studies of frontotemporal dementia suggest it has the shortest survival compared to other forms of dementia, and studies of Alzheimer's disease seem to report the longest survival periods. We have heard anecdotal discussions that people with young onset dementia deteriorate more quickly and survive for less time that people with late onset dementia, however the research suggests that the survival time is comparable for young onset and late onset dementia, if diagnosis is factored in (as frontotemporal dementia is more common in young onset cases).

The physical impact of dementia

We think of dementia as a brain disease. Since the brain controls the functions of the body (e.g. walking and coordination, breathing), dementia can also impact on physical function, and tends to do so later in the disease.

The following information on physical comorbidities of dementia is based on the research of Professor Sue Kurrle.

---

14 *https://fightdementia.org.au/sites/default/files/helpsheets*

Gait, balance and falls

Brain changes in dementia seem to affect coordination. The way that people walk (their gait) deteriorates in people with dementia (particularly dementia with Lewy bodies and vascular dementia). People with dementia can also experience loss of balance or feel unsteady on their feet (this is described by clinicians as postural instability). We discussed earlier the side effects of antipsychotic medications that may be prescribed to people with dementia relating to mobility and balance.

Changes in the way that visual information is processed by the brain, reduced self-awareness in physical abilities, reduced ability to concentrate and poorer ability to judge risk may also increase the chance of falling.

Of older people with dementia, 70-80% fall at least once a year — this is double the rate of other older people. Falls may result in injury, and fractures, including hip fractures, are three times more common in older people with dementia than other older people.

We know that we can decrease risk of falling in older people through a bundle of interventions which include:

> » Providing information on falls and falls risk, including in public places.
> » Making the home safer (an occupational therapist can help with this, and see dementia enabling environments in Chapter 7).
> » Choosing safe footwear — these are shoes which are flat or have low heels, have non-slip soles, fit well (so your foot shouldn't slide inside the shoe, and they shouldn't be too tight), completely surround the foot (so no slippers, sandals, or flip flops!) and support your feet.
> » Strength and balance exercises — such as practising going from sitting to standing and back down, exercises using a step (see a physiotherapist or occupational therapist for appropriate exercises for your body).
> » A medication review (some medications which impact on balance also increase risk of falls).

Researchers are currently testing whether these interventions decrease falls in people with dementia.

We can also take some precautions to prevent injury or complications if the person has a history of falls, including:

» Using hip protectors.

» Using a helmet.

» Installing a personal alarm or fall alarm — personal alarms are activated by the person themselves (by pressing a button on a device hung around the neck), and fall alarms detect that the person has fallen and send a notification to a monitoring centre.

Beyond evidence, the benefits of getting or keeping fit and strong by doing cardio, balance and strength exercises can only positively impact the risk of falls.

Epilepsy

Between 5 and 10% of people with dementia are reported to suffer from a seizure at least once — this is six times the rate in other older people. A seizure is caused by a sudden surge of electrical activity in the brain, and briefly affects how the person behaves. A seizure can involve the person losing consciousness or fainting, being confused, losing control of their body (e.g. falling, shaking, drooling, eye rolling, teeth clenching) and change their mood (e.g. sudden and unexplained anger, panic, joy or laughter).

It is important to know that seizures can occur, and can result in falls and unexpected behaviours. Report any possible seizures to your doctor. Recurring seizures may be treated with anticonvulsants.

Weight loss and malnutrition

Dementia appears to affect the energy balance in the body so that people with dementia are more likely to lose weight and this weight loss can start happening even before diagnosis. Dementia may also impact on how people with dementia interpret the signals from their stomach to their brain, which usually tell us that we are hungry, and some people with dementia forget to eat (though others forget that they have eaten and keep eating and eating!). Many people with dementia have a dulled sense of smell and taste and this may impact on how much they eat too. Many will also lose 10% of their body weight through the course of the disease, however a small proportion gain weight. If the person is overweight, then they may not be worried about weight loss, however this may be unhealthy weight loss if the person is losing muscle mass.

People with dementia are also more likely to be malnourished — this may be because they are eating less, or choosing less healthy foods. One person with dementia said, 'I don't get hungry any more, and I forget if I have eaten, so I'll either get very fat or very thin!' She lives alone, and this is a real issue for her and anyone living at home on their own with dementia. People with dementia living in nursing homes are twice as likely to be malnourished as other residents. If the person with dementia has lost more than 5% of their body weight in the last three-to-six months, then speak to your doctor. Interventions will depend on the reasons for the weight loss. These may include:

- nutritional supplements
- regular exercise
- if living alone at home, providing healthy meals, reminders to eat, and company for meals
- providing delicious food that the person likes, and making it visually appealing
- providing food that is culturally appropriate, or the person may not be willing to eat it even if they are really hungry
- making sure that the food is easy for the person to eat — for people with dementia who are having trouble eating with a fork and knife, provide finger foods
- making sure that the person is drinking enough water to avoid dehydration and reduce the occurrence of urinary tract infections, which are also symptomatic of dementia.

Maggie Beer's Appetite for Life foundation https://www. maggiebeerfoundation.org.au/ has a mission to improve the food experiences in aged care homes. Her website also includes tips and recipes for healthy eating.

Frailty

People with dementia become more frail — they lose strength, energy, and slow down. The frailty which comes with dementia may be because frailty and dementia share risk factors such as heart disease. Or frailty could be caused by the dementia. It may also be caused by factors such as the person not having been supported to continue to exercise regularly, or by changes in their diet.

However, physical exercise and rehabilitation (including strength and balance exercises) may reduce this risk, and are beneficial for everyone, not just people with dementia (discussed in Chapter 3). Improved nutrition may also help combat or reduce frailty.

Delirium

Dementia is the strongest risk factor for delirium. People with dementia are five times more likely to have delirium than other people their age. Delirium is a condition which starts rapidly and the person can be confused, disoriented and not be thinking or behaving in a way that is normal for them. If the person with dementia has rapid behavioural or mood changes — over a few hours or days, suspect delirium before you worry about the changes being caused by their dementia. Often delirium is not recognised in people with dementia.

The five main causes (5 Ps) of delirium are:
- poo — constipation
- pee — dehydration, urinary retention
- pus — infection
- pain — untreated pain
- pills — side effects of medication.

If you suspect delirium, seek immediate medical help from your doctor or emergency department. The causes of delirium are treatable, and once addressed, the symptoms will subside.

Dental health

Studies have suggested that poor dental health, tooth loss and gum disease are linked to dementia. We don't know if having dental problems causes dementia, or are a result of having dementia. People with dementia may have trouble with their dental health because:

> » They have less saliva in the mouth, either because of the disease or because of medications they are taking which cause dry mouth. Saliva fights germs in the mouth, and helps prevent bad breath, tooth decay and gum disease, and protects tooth enamel.
> » They forget to brush their teeth or do not brush their teeth properly.
> » Their diet has changed and they are eating more sugary foods.

For information about dental care see the section in Chapter 9 on dental care and dementia.

Urinary tract infections

Many people with dementia worry about becoming incontinent and drink less, hoping to alleviate the need to go to the toilet. This can increase the likelihood of getting urinary tract infections and these also take longer to be recognised in people with dementia.

Urinary tract infections are caused by bacteria in the urethra, bladder or kidneys. An untreated urinary tract infection can also cause delirium (see above), which can worsen the symptoms of dementia. Common symptoms of urinary tract infections include:

- frequently feeling the need to urinate, this may be urgent
- pain, or burning when urinating
- feeling like the bladder is still full after urinating
- pain above the pubic bone
- blood in the urine.

Please note that people can have urinary tract infections without any of the symptoms listed above, instead they may suddenly start to behave unusually or be very moody. If you suspect a urinary tract infection, see your doctor as soon as possible. Antibiotics are usually prescribed for UTIs.

Pneumonia

Pneumonia is a viral or bacterial infection of the lungs. In people with pneumonia, little sacs in the lungs called alveoli fill with pus and fluids, which interfere with breathing. It can be hard to tell the difference between symptoms of pneumonia and a cold, cough or flu. Common symptoms of pneumonia include:

- fever — with or without the chills
- cough
- chest pain
- rapid breathing
- breathing difficulties
- general tiredness and feeling of being sick
- loss of appetite
- abdominal pain
- headache.

If you suspect the person with dementia has pneumonia, see your doctor immediately. Treatment usually involves antibiotics and hydration. People with end-stage dementia often get pneumonia — and this is frequently the ultimate cause of death. For people with severe dementia with pneumonia, studies suggest that antibiotics prolong the person's life, but do not make them more comfortable in terms of pain, shortness of breath or fear. At this stage of dementia, the person may need to be moved to hospital for treatment, as antibiotics may need to be administered intravenously, and the person may need to be restrained to stop them from pulling the drip out. A choice families may have to make is whether to move a person with dementia to hospital for antibiotic treatment, and whether the stress of the move and hospital environment is worth prolonging the person's life.

This situation is one that you may wish to consider making an advanced care directive about (see Chapter 5 on Planning Ahead), even if you don't have dementia.

Management of other medical conditions

The impact of dementia on the person's ability to communicate about and manage their health can also exacerbate or complicate other physical illnesses such as diabetes, chronic obstructive pulmonary disorder, musculoskeletal disorders and cardiovascular disease. Some people with dementia and their families report experiencing a lack of active management or even concern for other health issues, once they have been diagnosed with dementia, and we recommend you actively seek whole of health support.

Quality of life vs length of life

Many people think that people with moderate-to-severe dementia will have poor quality of life. This is not necessarily the case. We moderate our expectations for our quality of life based on our circumstances and in comparison to others around us — this may be why older people tend to rate their quality of life higher than younger people, despite having more physical health difficulties.

Interestingly, people with dementia tend to rate their own quality of life more highly than the ratings made by aged care staff looking after them and much more highly than family ratings of quality of life.

In part, this may be why the public labelling of people with dementia (by people without dementia) as the ones suffering, is now being questioned so much and so publicly by people with dementia. Watching someone deteriorate and die is often far more difficult than for the person it is happening to.

One lady whose husband died from dementia said, 'It was hideous watching him deteriorate…to lose his ability to function and even swallow, and then die from starvation; but that was his wish. Watching this was more difficult for me than for him — he told me that he was so sorry. I had to go through it (watching him die), and said it was okay for him.'

We believe that we should be striving to give people with dementia good quality of life, rather than trying to prolong their life without thinking about quality. This person's story also highlights that it is often harder for the care partner than the person with the dementia, particularly towards the end of life.

New treatments and even a cure?

With the ageing of the world's populations, dementia is a growing health and economic issue internationally. Governments around the world have been investing funding and energy into working to develop a cure for dementia or a disease-altering treatment by 2025. The majority of research effort will be in relation to Alzheimer's disease. The pharmaceutical industry has already invested billions in research with little return — no new drugs have reached the market in the last 14 years. The number of pharmaceutical-sponsored human trials appears to have slowed down in recent years.

Current research in medications for treatment and prevention are targeting people early in the course of the disease. There has been discussion that many trials have failed because we treated people too late in the disease progress. For instance, we know that changes in the brain can occur decades before the first symptoms. So neuroimaging is being used to identify people without symptoms but with brain indicators of the disease (beta amyloid in the brain that can be detected using neuroimaging), and/or with genetic markers (apolipoprotein e4 variant) that place them at higher risk of Alzheimer's disease.

Given how long it takes to develop and test drugs, it is unlikely that any new drugs will come to market in the next five years; hopefully they will be available by 2025.

Chapter 5

PLANNING AHEAD

This chapter aims to help people with dementia and their care partner (if they have one), as well as their families, better understand the legal issues they may be faced with, and better understand their legal rights and the actions that can be taken to protect them. One of the greatest challenges we all face in life is coming to terms with death and dying, especially when the prospect is brought into focus after a diagnosis of any terminal illness, including dementia.

Too often, when diagnosed with any terminal illness, we have not planned for this part of our life. Many of us have never before thought about or discussed with our family our wishes about sickness and dying. When diagnosed with dementia, it is eminently important, if you are the person diagnosed with dementia, that you do think about what you want to happen in the future, as at some stage, it is very likely you will lose your cognitive and legal capacity to make your own choices about your lifestyle and health matters.

'...if a good death is the conclusion of a good life then it has to be a priority.' (Swaffer, 2016[15])

The late Dr Richard Taylor, a psychologist from Texas who was diagnosed with younger onset dementia, said many times, 'You are not

---

15 K Swaffer, What the Hell Happened to my Brain?: Living Beyond Dementia, *Jessica Kingsley Publishers, UK, 2016*

any closer to death than you were the day before you were diagnosed.' This is absolutely accurate, and it is important here to remind ourselves, as Kate often says, 'We are all born with a death sentence.'

Death and dying is the final part of one's life, and being told we may have a more finite time to live can be devastating, but it can also be seen as a gift, in that it makes us think very deeply about our own lives. It may help you to live more deeply, to live every day as if it is your last, just in case it is. It may also help your care partner and families to seek to only see the good in each other, and in situations and events and to let go of the petty disagreements we all have occasionally. It certainly helps many people stop 'sweating the small stuff' so often.

A diagnosis of a terminal illness makes us feel temporary, transient, and somehow perishable; mortal. Facing up to the fact that dementia is a terminal illness is made more difficult because the focus will be more on our own quality of life being compromised, on not living fully functionally, and not being in a position to make our own choices.

The idea of not knowing who our family and friends are, or not recognising ourselves in a mirror, makes it very daunting, and colours the reality of the illness. This makes it hard to make end-of-life decisions in a timely fashion. We can spend too much time worrying about what capacity or function will become impaired, rather than focusing on the important things like how we want to be treated when our capacity declines, and how we might wish to die.

Those of you living with dementia should embrace, and make sure others embrace the phrase 'nothing about us, without us', especially when it comes to your end of life wishes.

If you don't speak up while you still can for what you want, then when you are incapacitated you will place a significant burden and responsibility on others as they will have to make difficult choices for you; most often these are the very people whom you love the most.

If you don't make your wishes clear, then you may not be provided with the end of life care you would have chosen yourself. For example, ask yourself, do you wish to be kept alive in the late stages of dementia (or after a stroke or serious accident) by a feeding tube and intravenous infusion, when you may not be able to swallow enough to drink and eat?

The information here may include issues that you have not previously considered or discussed with anyone else, and whilst this may seem like a lot of information to digest, and it may be helpful to review this chapter over a period of time. It is important for you to discuss your views and wishes with your family and friends, and finalise relevant documents while you are still legally capable of doing so. There are also services available to support you through this process, if you need them. Of course, your situation and life is unique to you, so what is important to someone else, may not be to you. It is your life, and ultimately it is your death.

The information provided here is of a general nature only; we recommend you seek legal advice if you feel you need support with planning and making these types of decisions.

As Australia has a federal system of government, there may be some areas of law that are governed by Federal laws, and others that are governed by State or Territory laws. The important thing is to be clear on what the law is in your State/Territory, and how it is administered.

More information about planning ahead can be obtained by contacting the Alzheimer's Australia National Dementia Helpline on 1800 100 500, or by visiting their Talk2Me website http://start2talk.org.au

Managing money and administrative affairs

Managing money becomes problematic for people with dementia as the disease progresses. A number of difficulties will surface, including things like seeing numbers back to front, problems with simple math, being unable to do calculations any more, and so on. Even recognising how much a note or coin is worth may be a problem. At some stage, almost every person diagnosed with dementia will require help to manage day-to-day money matters. It is easy to spend money even without dementia, but add in a diagnosis of dementia, and it can become very problematic. This section is written with more of a focus on the person with dementia, but will help everyone facing dementia in his or her family.

One person with dementia said:

> I had only been diagnosed for a couple of years, and one day, ordered
> $750 worth of wine. When the wine was delivered three days

later, I had no recollection of the purchase. We certainly had a great
Christmas that year, but after that, we had to change my access to the
accounts, and get a credit card with a smaller balance.

Giving up your independence and freedom in money matters can be emotionally difficult, just like giving up your driver's license. Therefore, it will help to sort out day-to-day money matters and suggest arrangements for the future as soon as possible.

Some care partners have never had any involvement in managing the finances. Having to take over from the person with dementia can be not only emotionally difficult, but hard work. It can mean you will need to place more trust in people like accountants, financial advisors, family members, and sometimes even friends. For example, one man had never taken money out of a bank or paid a bill in his whole life until after his wife died, so, at the age of about 70, he had to learn to do these things. He had not ever even taken money out of an ATM, so this was a huge task, and one that quickly became too much for him.

Here are some things that may help you manage your financial and administrative affairs if you are a person living with dementia:

» Giving someone you trust access to your online banking accounts (they will require passwords).
» Getting help paying bills — this might be helped by setting up automatic payments with regular providers.
» Making a list of your passwords for the many accounts you have with different organisations (e.g. Centrelink, health fund, insurance fund); there is software you can use for this called Dashlane and it is very helpful for storing passwords, as well as providing you with passwords with a very high security rating. See the resource list for the details.
» Find an accountant that you trust, and ensure you have appointed someone legally to assist in managing your financial affairs (see Power of Attorney below) if you need support doing it, or can no longer do it for yourself.

Memory Banc is an organisation set up by Kay Bransford in the USA, who was the main care partner for her mother and father, who both had dementia. She has developed a number of tools and resources through her own experience and challenges of having to take over her parent's financial and legal affairs.

On her website[16] which we have listed in the resource list, she says:

> *When my parents had trouble remembering how to manage the chequebook, or even where the chequebook was, I stepped in to assist them. They had Wills, a Trust and the Power of Attorney was done, but that doesn't really help you when you need to manage the day-to-day affairs.*

There are some free downloads on her site, and the section, 'What Documents Should I Protect?' is an excellent resource.

Wills

A will is a document which legally sets out your wishes after your death including how your assets are going to be distributed, who is going to care for any dependents, establishment of trusts, funeral arrangements and who you want to be the executor (the person who deals with all the paperwork in relation to your estate including settling debts and gathering and distributing assets) and trustee (the person who administers any trusts set up in the will).

If you die without a will, a government formula is used to divide your assets between your family; this formula differs by state.

One son said, 'It was a bloody nightmare my father not having a will, it took years to sort things out for mum.'

Most people use a lawyer or solicitor to write their wills, though legally this is not required. When preparing to make a will — make a list of your assets including property, cash, vehicles, investments and superannuation. You may also want to make a list of items with sentimental value that you want to pass on to specific people.

The law about wills in Australia is different in each state and territory.

---

16   *http://www.memorybanc.com*

State-specific information is available at www.australia.gov.au — search wills.

Enduring Power of Attorney

A Power of Attorney is a document, which legally appoints someone to look after your affairs under specific circumstances for example, when you're going away on a holiday or when you're going to be in hospital. When you appoint a Power of Attorney, you give that attorney the legal authority to look after your legal and financial affairs on your behalf such as selling or renting out your property, paying bills and taxes, and investing your money. In some states in Australia such as Queensland and Victoria, a Power of Attorney can also deal with personal, medical and lifestyle decisions such as deciding where you will live, and what services and medical treatment you will receive. In other states such as New South Wales, an Enduring Guardian needs to be appointed to make lifestyle decisions.

Appointing an Enduring Power of Attorney will give that attorney the authority to make ongoing decisions for you after you have lost your capacity to make decisions. The attorney must accept the appointment in writing before using their authority.

Choose someone to be your power of attorney that you trust to act in your best interests, and who will manage your financial and legal affairs in a responsible manner. It is important to ask the person whether he/she is happy to act as an enduring power of attorney before making the appointment. If your affairs are complex, then you need to choose someone who will be able to cope with the task. You can choose to appoint more than one attorney, and if you appoint more than one, then decide how the attorneys can make decisions. For example, you could require that the attorneys make decisions jointly and both sign any document, or you could allow them to make decisions individually so that only one attorney is required to decide and sign a document.

The law about Enduring Power of Attorney in Australia is different in each state and territory. State-specific information is available at www.australia.gov.au — search Powers of Attorney.

Enduring guardianship

An Enduring Guardian is someone you appoint to make personal, medical and lifestyle decisions for you when you have lost capacity to make these decisions. In some states an Enduring Power of Attorney can include the same powers as an Enduring Guardianship. An Enduring Guardian can make on your behalf personal, medical and lifestyle decisions such as where you will live, and what services and medical treatment you will receive.

Ms J said when we were talking to her about this topic, 'I want to die peacefully, and without someone shoving a tube in me to force feed me, so I guess I'd better get that stuff sorted!'

Her partner had just said she would not want her partner to die (quite naturally so), so without this type of document in place, would probably ask the doctors and nurses to 'intervene'.

Choose someone you trust to be able to make good decisions according to your values and wishes to be your Enduring Guardian. It is important to ask the person whether he/she is happy to act as an enduring guardian before making the appointment. You can give your guardian directions about how to exercise the decision-making powers (e.g. to take into account the wishes of other family members before making decisions).

We have talked to people who felt emotionally unable to carry out the person's wishes to be allowed to die without interventions, so it is perhaps the most important decision you will make when choosing someone to carry out your end of life wishes. One other thing to consider is your age, as if you are retired, possibly many of your friends and family are as well, and you might need to choose more than one person to allow for the fact they might be travelling overseas when decisions like this need to be made.

The law about Enduring Guardianship in Australia is different in each state and territory. State-specific information is available at www.australia. gov.au — search Powers of Attorney.

Advanced care planning and advance care directives

An advance care directive is a written document that provides information about your wishes, values, and any treatments you would not wish to receive when you are no longer able to make these choices or express these preferences. The document is both to inform health care workers, and help your Enduring Power of Attorney or Guardian, or family and friends make decisions on your behalf. Advance care directives are often discussed as being in relation to end of life care or terminal care, but this is not necessarily so. Advance care directives can apply to any aspect of your life when you can no longer make your own decisions.

Advance care planning is the process of talking with your health care workers, medical Power of Attorney or Enduring Guardian, family and friends about issues around your future health care wishes. It can prevent future conflict between family and friends who might disagree on what the best course of treatment is.

> *I know my family will fight over everything (sigh), not just the money when I'm dead, but about what they think I would want when I'm heading out the door [he meant deteriorating and can't make his own decision]...I know I should get these things in writing, to stop the fights and make sure they do what I want. And they probably won't believe this, but I'd rather go into a home, than live with them if I get to that stage, you know, when I can't look after myself. (Man with dementia)*

Advanced care directives often specify the conditions under which you may not want specific treatments. The treatments that you may choose not to be treated with are cardiopulmonary resuscitation (CPR — to keep your heart pumping when it has stopped), assisted ventilation (a machine to help you breathe), artificial hydration and nutrition (a tube into your stomach or into a vein), surgery, antibiotics or any treatment that may obstruct your natural dying. Conditions under which you may have treatment withheld are: if you have a terminal, incurable, or irreversible illness or condition, if you are in a persistent vegetative state, if you are permanently unconscious, or if you are so seriously ill or injured that you are unlikely to recover to the extent that you can survive without the continued use of life-sustaining measures. These conditions are somewhat subjective, and those people making decisions on your behalf may still have to interpret whether the situation fits your wishes.

It can be difficult to anticipate how your future self would make a decision when the real situation arises. For instance, you might feel now that you wouldn't want to stay alive if you were constantly experiencing a lot of pain. However, in the event of living in that situation, you may feel that even with the pain, there is still a lot that is valuable and enjoyable in your life and you do want to live.

As well as discussing these issues with your enduring power of attorney/ guardian and family and friends, it is really helpful to talk to your doctor or health care worker as part of advanced care planning. This is so that you're well in formed in understanding the conditions and treatments that you're listing and their consequences. You don't need to talk to a lawyer to draw up an advanced care directive.

For more information and advanced care planning tools see Advanced Care Planning Australia: www.advancecareplanning.org.au

Advanced Care Directives SA

From 1 July 2014, the *Advance Care Directives Act 2013* came into play in South Australia, as well as changes to the *Consent to Medical Treatment and Palliative Care Act 1995* and the *Guardianship and Administration Act 1993*. This changes who can consent to or refuse healthcare on a patient's behalf, so it is important that we all have some understanding of what this means for us.

Key points:

> » There is an Advance Care Directive Form on which a
>   person can appoint a substitute decision-maker and/or
>   write instructions about their future healthcare, and their
>   wishes for their living arrangements and personal matters.
> » This Advance Care Directive applies at any time that the
>   patient has impaired decision-making capacity in relation
>   to the decision — not just at end of life.
> » A key principle of these changes is that everyone making
>   decisions for a patient with impaired decision-making
>   capacity must act as if 'they are in the patient's shoes'
>   and make decisions as they would have done in the same
>   circumstances. This is the case whether or not the patient

has an Advance Care Directive.

» A refusal of treatment, which is relevant to the situation, must be complied with (binding refusal).

» Wherever possible, a patient's wishes and values should be complied with as appropriate (non-binding requests).

» There are protections for those complying with an ACD in good faith and without negligence.

» There are protections for providing health care against a refusal of health care but only when acting in urgent and uncertain emergencies.

» There is no requirement to provide treatment that will not benefit the patient in the terminal phase of an illness.

» There is a clear hierarchy of who to obtain consent from when a patient's decision-making capacity is impaired. Enduring Power of Guardianship, Anticipatory Directions and Medical Power of Attorney still have legal effect, which means the protections apply. But there are some changes in how these apply. The new Advance Care Directive form, if the patient has one, supersedes any pre-existing forms.

» There is a simplified dispute resolution process that is provided by the Public Advocate (24/7) should disputes not be resolved at the hospital or health service.

» An Advance Care Directive cannot be used to demand health care and for anything illegal such as euthanasia, assisted suicide or refusal of mandatory treatment such as mental health orders.

For more information, visit: www.advancecaredirectives.sa.gov.au

Mental capacity and decision-making

What does capacity to make decisions really mean and why is it important? This is an important question to consider, even if you don't have dementia.

Any of us may become incapacitated, whether by dementia or an unexpected medical condition such as a stroke or accident, and may need someone else to make decisions about our life, and in particular our end of life, if we have not made them ourselves. If you have not planned for this, then how you are treated, whether you are kept alive by a respirator or some other medical intervention, and how you die, may not be the way you wish.

I'd hate XX to have any say in my care! We've never got on so I don't think she'd respect my wishes, but she is the one they all listen to since she was a nurse, and her husband is an accountant so they'd probably want to manage my money as well as my health. (Lady with dementia)

For the person diagnosed with dementia, it is really important to consider what might happen at the point where you no longer have the capacity to make your own decisions. The legislation across Australia is based on the international principle of 'presumption of capacity'. This means that you are assumed to have capacity to make your own decisions unless someone can prove that you do not, and this cannot happen just because a family member or non-professional person claims that you no longer have capacity. Capacity is decision-specific, so even if you have been diagnosed with dementia, you may still have capacity to make all or at least some of your own decisions, especially if you have been diagnosed with dementia in the early phase of the disease. Decision-making capacity may also fluctuate significantly over time and depend on the context, such as the time of day, location, noise, stress or anxiety levels, medication, or infection.

Please remember that in Australia, the legislation regarding a person's capacity to make his or her own decisions differs in each state or territory. Some documents may also only be valid in your own state, although this is changing.

Can I still be involved in decision-making if I no longer have capacity?

The person who has been appointed to make a decision on your behalf should continue to involve you in the decision-making process to the extent you are able. People sometimes also take part in supported decision-making. Supported decision-making is a term that has arisen from concerns about the lack of involvement between a substitute decision-maker and the person they are making decisions for.

It is a more inclusive, consultative and shared way of making decisions that is generally viewed as being more in line with a person's legal and human rights. Supported decision-making may be based on a formal agreement, or an informal network of people who support you to achieve your individual goals and decisions that are based on your own needs, views and wishes.

Who makes the ruling I no longer have capacity to make my own decisions?

One older man asked, 'Can my son or daughter just decide I no longer have capacity and force me to go into a home and take over all of my affairs?'

The arbitration about your capacity to make decisions for yourself is based on evidence, and in most cases will require a report from a health professional, for example your doctor or psychologist. There are a variety of tests that these professionals are likely to use to assess your capacity, and to guide them in their ruling about your capacity to make your own decisions.

'One of the biggest fears my older patients talk to me about is who will make decisions for them when they no longer have capacity, and who decides this.' (general practitioner)

Planning ahead, discussing your wishes with family members or close friends and appointing someone (and in some cases appointing more than one person is helpful) to make decisions for you if you do not have capacity will ensure that your wishes will be legally respected. If you do appoint more than one person to make your decisions for both financial and/or personal and health care matters, you will need to say how you want them to make their decisions. For example, you may want them to make the decisions jointly, which means that they do it together, so they need to agree, or you may say that they can do it severally, which means that any one of them can do it. We recommend you seek advice on this if you have any concerns about how decisions may be made.

If you have appointed someone to make decisions for you for a time in the future, when that person thinks that perhaps you now lack capacity, they can discuss it with your GP. However, they cannot simply make this decision on their own.

Also, people not legally appointed as your legal guardian or a supported decision-maker who have concerns about your decision-making capacity, can make an application to the relevant Board or Tribunal. The Board or Tribunal in your state will then decide whether you can make your own decisions, or whether someone else or a government agency needs to make them for you. The decision of the Board or Tribunal is reliant on reports from doctors, or other health professionals.

Appointing someone to make decisions for me when I am no longer able to make my own

While you still have legal capacity, you can choose to appoint someone to make decisions for you if, at some future time, you lack capacity to make your own decisions. This person is called a substitute decision-maker, and in many cases, people will choose more than one person. Whilst there are no laws that state that you have to appoint a substitute decision-maker, there are laws that state what will happen if you lose capacity and you have not appointed anyone to make financial, personal, and health decisions for you. While you still can, it is wise to make your own decisions and do your own planning, including appointing someone you know and trust to carry out your wishes. Sometimes members of the family do not agree on the decisions being made by the appointed decision-makers, and they can make an application to the relevant Board or Tribunal. Family mediation is usually offered at this point to assist families.

In Australia, each state and territory has a different system for the appointment of people or agencies to make decisions for you when you no longer have capacity to make your own decisions. They also often have different terminology when referring to the substitute decision-maker, and different rules about the types of decisions substitute decision-makers can make.

The term most often used throughout Australia to refer to substitute decision-makers appointed by you for financial matters is 'Attorney', and the term most often used to refer to substitute decision-makers appointed by you for personal and health care decisions is 'Enduring Guardian'.

For more information on all of these matters, and before seeking professional legal advice, which can be costly, you may wish to refer to the Alzheimer's Australia publication 'Understanding the Legal Rights of People with Dementia,'[17] which will give you much more detail on all of these matters.

We can never completely avoid conflict, but if you make your wishes clear, and legalise them through formalising them, then others will not have to argue about what your wishes were or are. Make sure that you don't just do the paperwork but talk to your families about what you want. Many families report that arguing about what is best for you or how they should interpret your wishes still goes on, even when you have made your wishes clear.

The benefits of doing this are significant and they are concrete things that can help to reduce conflict between loved ones, at a time when stress, anxiety and possible family or doctor conflicts are high. Your wishes can be clearly articulated, and this helps your family to understand what you want when, or if, you can no longer speak for yourself. Secondly, when there is an unexpected sudden health crisis and, for example, an ambulance needs to be called, the paramedics can be given the Directive as soon as they come and are then obliged to act in accordance with your wishes. There will be no grey areas about what you want.

Think about, and then make clear what YOUR wishes about YOUR future care needs and palliative care needs are. That way, no-one has to guess what your wishes are, reducing conflict amongst family or friends who are supporting you, and ensuring your health, lifestyle and end-of-life wishes are respected.

The really important thing to remember, whether you have dementia or not, is that if you don't make these decisions whilst you are still able to, someone will have to make them for you.

---

17 *https://fightdementia.org.au/sites/default/files/NATIONAL/documents/ Dementia-and-your-legal-rights.pdf*

Chapter 6

LIVING WITH A DIAGNOSIS OF DEMENTIA

This chapter will give you practical information and strategies to help you continue to live as well as possible, in spite of having dementia. It is difficult coming to terms with dementia, and even more so with living with the disAbilities it can cause, but that doesn't have to be a reason not to 'fight for your life', as you probably would if diagnosed with a terminal cancer.

Accepting you are disabled, if you have been a high functioning and able-bodied person is emotionally challenging, and initially can really affect your self-worth and self-esteem.

Managing the symptoms of dementia as disAbilities however, can enable you to live much more positively, independently and productively for longer.

One lady with dementia said; 'It is my responsibility while I still can, to tell people I have dementia and it has caused me to have many disabilities; otherwise, how can I reasonably expect them to support me if I don't tell them?'

Whilst it may be hard coming to terms with seeing dementia symptoms as disAbilities, it really is worth working on strategies to support them, and more fruitful to do so early after the diagnosis. It is not always possible to be continually living well (whatever that means to you) with dementia.

Sometimes it is almost too much to get out of bed. That's okay too, we all need to do that, or feel like that some days. Dementia certainly has its unique challenges that affect people in different ways, and it is also a progressive terminal illness where, ultimately, your functioning at almost all levels will require support.

Almost no-one likes failing, so setting up as many supports as you can will be helpful for staying positive and continuing to experience joy in your life.

Strategies to support cognitive disAbilities and memory loss

Staying active socially and continuing to be challenged physically and intellectually is the most positive pathway for people following a diagnosis of dementia. In Chapter 3 we discussed the reasons for staying active. We've also discussed how Prescribed Disengagement, coupled with the grief and loss that many people with dementia experience, can result in people diagnosed with dementia retreating from life.

We don't wish to imply that you HAVE to be busy doing things 100% of the time, or that if your dementia gets worse it's because you haven't been active enough. We're just suggesting that one way of positively managing the progression of the disease is to keep engaging with the world and living your life, as you would with any other disease or illness.

When we have disAbilities, it is important to develop approaches (we call them life enhancement strategies or aids) to overcome or manage them. If you'd sprained your ankle, you would use a crutch. In the same way, if we are forgetful, we use a list! You may have other cognitive disAbilities that would also benefit from strategies any other person with a disAbility would use to support them. It takes a little time, and sometimes experimentation, to figure out what strategies and supports work for you individually, and for each of your disAbilities.

With your disAbilities, you may have to use a metaphorical walking stick, a ramp, a lot of post it notes, and a safety rail. The strategies you choose will depend on your cognitive strengths. For instance, if you are good at taking notes and processing written instructions, then use these. If you have trouble reading, then you may choose to use visual instructions (i.e. pictures or photographs) and record information in audio files.

Here are some ideas for life enhancement strategies for a range of different disAbilities. They may or may not work in your circumstance, but trialling them may be useful. These ideas can also be adapted or implemented with the help of health care professionals, care partners and service providers. There are more life enhancement ideas under support for disAbilities in the dementia and employment section.

It is also important to remember that dementia is not only about memory loss and problem solving difficulties, many people also have sensory challenges as a result of dementia. Even if your eyesight is still perfect, you may experience vision changes that are due to changes in your visual perceptual abilities or spatial awareness. You may have hypersensitivity to noise, changes to taste and smell, changes to you interests such as music or hobbies, or you may experience hallucinations. We hope the next few pages of life enhancement strategies and aids will support you to live better with these disAbilities. Agnes Houston, a woman living with dementia from Scotland, has also produced a simple booklet about this, 'Dementia & Sensory Challenges', which you can find in the resource list.

Problems relating to memory
Problem: I forget to take my medication
Possible strategies:
>> Use an electronic reminder on your phone or pre-set an alarm clock.
>> Set up a system where others remind you in person or by phone.

Problem: I sometimes take my medication twice
Possible strategies:
> » Keep a list of all your medications including the dose, so it is easy to access this information, and for your care partner and any medical professionals to see.
> » Take photographs of the medications and make a visual schedule if this is helpful in taking the medication or filling your dosette box.
> » Set up a system for taking your medication — use a pill organisation or dosette box, or ask your pharmacist to put it into a Webster pack. This way you can more easily take the right medication at the right time, and you or others can see if you've missed a dose.

By way of example, we know of a lady with dementia who has set up a medication reminder on her phone and then her husband has a reminder set up on his phone 15 minutes later to call and see if the medication has been taken, then one of their adult children has a reminder 15 minutes later to remind her husband!

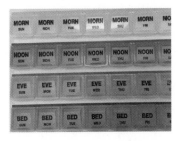
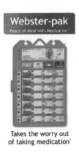

Takes the worry out
of taking medication

Problem: I can't keep track of appointments
Possible strategies:
> » Use a diary.
> » Use a large whiteboard in your home, with the appointments for the week set up each day or week.
> » Have someone you trust manage your appointments for you.
> » Arrange with everyone you have regular appointments with to phone you the day before, and the day of the

appointment, as a reminder.

» Many health professionals, and others such as hairdressers and beauticians now send a text message as a reminder the day before.

» Ask people you have regular appointments with to make sure you put the appointment in your diary, and also give the information to your care partner.

» Post-it notes assist in keeping track of things and sometimes work as reminders, including for appointments.

» Use laminated sheets, with the weekly plan of an activity.

One woman with dementia told us that after arriving at a medical appointment on the wrong day three times in a short space of time, her specialist then suggested to his secretary that she add the next appointment into the patient's diary, and also give a second appointment card for her next appointment to her husband. Most of the time, this works.

Weekly walking program

Program:

Mondays	Church walking group 10:30am	To be picked up by Mrs D
Tuesdays	Use walker at home	
Wednesdays	Walk with volunteer (Kate)	To depart from home at 11am
Thursdays	Norwood Walking Group (Heart foundation)	To be picked up by Mr J or Mrs P at 9am
Fridays	Walk with volunteer (Kate)	To depart from home at 9am

Note: Walks will be no longer than 30 minutes in the first week, but may increase depending on ability and desire.

Contact details of walkers:

Walking with:	Contact numbers:
Mrs D (Sophia)	
Kate	
Mr J (Dave)	
Mrs P (Janice)	
Two copies placed near back door, and in kitchen	

Problem: I can't remember people's names

Possible strategies:

> » The use of social media is really helpful, for those people who are on social media. For example, Facebook automatically includes pictures of people who are messaging or posting, which can work well as prompts.

> » Use errorless learning or spaced retrieval strategies to help you learn names (see below for more details).

> » Ask colleagues (if still working) and friends and family to add their profile image into their email footer is helpful if you use emails to communicate.

> » Ask anyone who sends you things in the post to add a small photo of themselves and include their Christian and surnames on the back of the envelope so it can support you better in remembering them.

> » Have a set of laminated photos, or a small photo album with photos and the names of those you meet with often — you can flip through this before going to a social event

> » Ask your care partner or a person you often attend social activities with to remind you of names as you arrive.

> » Ask the person you've forgotten to remind you what their name is. This is emotionally challenging as you may feel embarrassed not knowing the names of family and friends. It is especially so when you meet up with people you 'know you know', but still can't remember their name.

Errorless learning is a strategy where you don't have to make mistakes when you learn something (in contrast with trial and error). The principles of errorless learning are to practise the information you want to learn repeatedly without guessing, and to support the learning using cues. You would start with photos of the people with their name written next to it — don't do too many of these, three to five may be enough. Go over these photos saying the names out loud — practise these at least five times. Then write a 'clue' to the person's name on a post-it note — this could be 'starts with P' or 'rhymes with Sob', or 'a type of flower'. Cover up the person's name with the post-it clue. Go through the photos, and if the clue doesn't help you to remember the person's name, then look at their name underneath. Don't guess. Once you can remember the names with the help of the clues and you've done this five times over, cover the clues up with blank sticky notes. Once again try and remember the person's name, and if you can't, don't guess, use the clue. If that doesn't help, check the name. You can find more information about errorless learning on YouTube.

Spaced retrieval is a learning technique where you recall the information that you're trying to learn at increasingly greater intervals. So if you're trying to learn two important new names, you would try and remember them after 1 minute, 2 minutes, 4 minutes, 8 minutes, 16 minutes, 32 minutes…as long as you need. Set an alarm to remind yourself to think about the new names. If you can't remember the names at each time point, then look them up, and go back to a shorter interval (e.g. if you couldn't remember at 4 minutes, try again after 2 minutes and then 4 minutes). Errorless learning and spaced retrieval strategies can be used together.

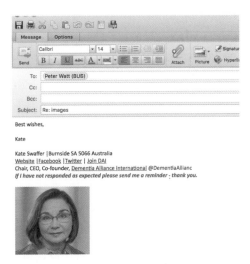

Best wishes,

Kate

Kate Swaffer | Burnside SA 5066 Australia
Website | Facebook | Twitter | Join DAI
Chair, CEO, Co-founder, Dementia Alliance International @DementiaAllianc
If I have not responded as expected please send me a reminder - thank you.

Problem: I keep forgetting to do things (like taking my glasses or walking stick)

Possible strategies:

» Develop regular routines and predictable schedules, allowing you more of a chance to function on autopilot.

» Have family or friends support you with verbal or phone call reminders.

» Use lists (you can laminate them if you use them often). For example, use a laminated sheet with the sequence of what to do in the bathroom and when getting dressed, have a laminated sheet with all the things to pack when you travel and a laminated sheet at the front door with what to take when you go out.

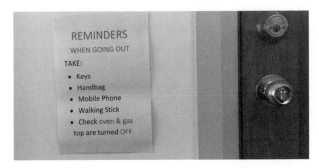

Problem: I keep forgetting to take my house keys with me when I go out

Possible strategies:

> » Have a laminated list near the front door to remind you of things to take with you when you go out.
> » Get a key safe fitted outside your home.
> » Leave a key with a neighbour who is at home a lot.
> » Attach a spare key inside your handbag, or keep a spare in your wallet.
> » If you go out often with the same people, leave a spare key with them and ask them to keep it in their handbag/wallet or car.

Problem: I keep forgetting to turn off the oven or cooktop

Possible strategies:

> » Stop cooking when home alone.
> » If you forget to do that, try using a laminated notice either posted onto the wall next to the oven, or on top of the cooker (see image below).
> » Install a device that automatically turns off your stove — there are versions that turn off after a set time (e.g. 30 minutes), and others with a motion detector that turn off if you're not standing in front of the cooker.
> » Set up a routine with your care partner or a family member or friend to help you cook things once or twice a week and then set up your meals to store in either the fridge or freezer.
> » Start a weekly cooking group in your own home with friends, asking them to support you by cooking in bulk together, and putting things in the freezer; this can be a hugely fun way of not only not burning the house down, but having meals prepared. This could be doubly helpful, as there will also be many days your care partner will feel too tired to cook, if they have taken over most of this necessary activity, and also means you don't miss out on cooking if that was something you loved doing.

» Place a laminated sheet at the front door with a note to check the oven and cook top is off (See image above for 'I keep forgetting to do things').

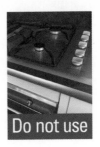

Do not use

Problem: I keep getting lost, even within my own home
Possible strategies:
» Get an app for directions on your phone and learn how to use it, if possible.
» At home and in other places where you spend a lot of time, place laminated signs in areas where you get confused (e.g. where there are many doors leading off the same hallway, or the bathroom) — sometimes having a picture of what is in the room is helpful as well as writing in a bold clear font what the room is (black text on white paper or card is the most dementia enabling).
» Let people you spend time with know that you have trouble with finding your way and ask for their help; try not feel embarrassed about it.
» If going to a new place where you think you will get lost, prepare by printing a map or floor plan (e.g. of a shopping centre) and planning the route.
» If going into a big shopping centre, take a photo with your phone of the entrance you used.
» If you are still driving, take a photo of where you park the car, including which floor.
» Ask for directions rather than getting frustrated at being lost
» Wear a 'safe return' bracelet, available from Alzheimer's Australia in most states. Some people with dementia find this bracelet humiliating and won't wear it, as it is not discreet in the same way a medic alert bracelet is. If this is the case, use one of the other strategies listed here.

» Carry a card that has your personal details including your address, and contact numbers for your care partner or someone who will be able to help you get home.

Signs as visual aids:

Contrast of area before and after placement of signs visual aids:

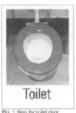

Toilet

Fig. 1 Sign for toilet door

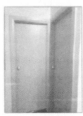

Fig. 1 Appearance before placement of signs

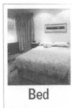

Bed

Fig. 2 Sign for bedroom

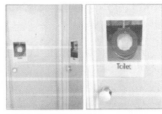

Fig. 2 Appearance after placement of signs

Problem: I keep forgetting important information

Possible strategies:

» Use your writing skills to keep notes or use a journal.

» Use the camera on your phone, or another camera, to take visual reminders.

» Record the information onto your phone or computer — make sure you (or someone else) label the recordings well so you can find the information you need.

» Ask others to support you by attending important appointments or meetings with you and taking notes for you.

» Always keep a small notebook and a pen with you, or purchase a Boogie Board (a small, electronic whiteboard).

» Record your visits to doctors or other important things you need to be able to recall at a later time.

Problem: I have trouble finding the right words
Possible strategies:

» Practise recalling items, events and people you have trouble with (you may keep a list of words that you commonly forget). Use written, picture, photo or auditory exercises to help you with this, and practice saying those words and phrases.
» Label things around your home.
» Talk about the meaning of the word if you can't remember the actual word, and let others provide the word if it helps the conversation continue.
» Ask others to wait and give you time.
» Spend an hour a day practicing word recall.
» Ask others to slow down.
» Come back to it later; it might come back to you.
» Others prompting you can sometimes make it harder, so ask them not to unless you ask them for help.

Problems relating to attention, concentration and problem solving

Problem: I am easily distracted
Possible strategies:

» Make an effort to focus on a task, and keep refocusing — this can be done by taking notes of where you are up to.
» Use step-by-step guides.
» Use a whiteboard for the things you want to get done throughout a day, with step-by-step guides for each task or activity so you have somewhere to refer back to.
» Give yourself longer to do things.

Problem: I lose concentration during conversations
Possible strategies:

» Where possible, plan to have important appointments or meetings at times when you are at your best (e.g. in the morning). If this is not possible, then try and make sure that you're well rested before the meeting.

- » For important conversations (e.g. doctor's appointments) prepare a list of questions or discussion points.
- » Ask for important information to be written down, and take brochures if they are available.
- » Ask if you can record important conversations on your phone or iPad, so you can go back and listen to them later; SoundNote is a helpful app for this, especially if you want to take notes as well as record a conversation or meeting.
- » Try and have one conversation at a time, and when multiple conversations are happening, focus all of your attention on one and, if possible, take the conversation somewhere you won't be distracted.
- » Ask the other person to repeat themselves, and try not to feel embarrassed about asking them.
- » Ask for other noise to be minimised if possible.
- » You might decide it is easier to make an excuse and leave the conversation or group e.g. go to the bathroom, or if at home, say you are going to have a rest, even if you simply go and watch TV, listen to music or read a book.
- » Apologise and wait until your thoughts come around to the subject again. They may or may not, but try not to get upset as you are the one with dementia; most will be very understanding if they know you have disAbilities.

Problem: I find myself confused about what I'm meant to be doing half way through something

Possible strategies:

- » Use lists to remind you, and so others also know what you want to do.
- » Ask others to help keep you on track.
- » Try not to worry about it, many people, even those without dementia, get distracted.
- » Make prompt sheets for common tasks that you get confused with. For example, Kate uses this prompt sheet for making a coffee.

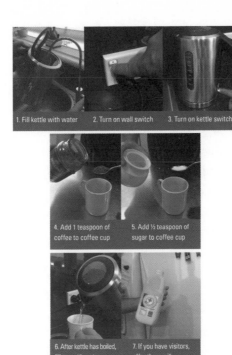

1. Fill kettle with water 2. Turn on wall switch 3. Turn on kettle switch
4. Add 1 teaspoon of coffee to coffee cup 5. Add ½ teaspoon of sugar to coffee cup
6. After kettle has boiled, fill cup with water 7. If you have visitors, offer them milk

Problem: It takes me a long time and a lot of effort to make decisions, even about small things such as what to wear in the morning

Possible strategies:

> » Ask for help planning your wardrobe or other things you have trouble making decisions on.
> » Rearrange and declutter your wardrobe, for example place all of the summer clothes into another wardrobe during winter, make sure tops and trousers are together, and so on.
> » Ask your care partner or support person to lay out your clothes each day, in the order you need to put them on; even having a laminated help sheet can be useful, e.g. the order, starting with your underwear, if that has become more difficult.
> » Wear the same things a lot — this means having more than one of the things you most like to wear.
> » Sometimes, using a wall calendar or chart, and making

plans on it gives you visual cues for the day or week. Kate even adds things like doing the washing.

» When going shopping, write on your list the exact number of items (e.g. three tomatoes) or brand you use to reduce the number of decisions you need to make at the shop.

One man said to us, 'I only want to wear brown and black now, so don't bother buying me anything else. I have no idea why my wife does! And I'm the one with dementia.' [Rolled his eyes, with a cheeky grin.]

Some people with dementia will become fixated on some things; if it is clothing, it really doesn't matter if they wear the same things repeatedly, hence the value of buying a few of the same.

Problem: It takes me a long time to do things, much longer than it used to
Possible strategies:

» Develop regular routines and predictable schedules, that way you can more easily run on autopilot.

» If you can, accept that some things will take longer and have realistic expectations.

» Use instruction lists, such as the coffee making instructions pictured above.

» Try not to set unrealistic goals that will set you up for failure.

» Give up doing some things and let someone else do them — this may be difficult emotionally, as most of us are very independent.

One younger man said, 'Well, I don't fly planes, and now doing the books [accounts] feels like that, so why not let someone else do them?!'

Problem: I have trouble knowing what order to do things
Possible strategies:

» Ask someone to work alongside you, so you can copy the sequencing of a task, e.g. when setting the table or hanging out the washing

» Use laminated lists (e.g. of how to make a cup of tea or coffee, with visuals), as shown above

Problems related to processing visual information

Problem: I am having difficulty reading as the lines and words get mixed up

Possible strategies:

» Get your eyesight tested, but note it is often nothing to do with eyesight.

» Hire or buy audio books.

» Laminate a coloured sheet the size of the things you read regularly, with a cut out in it the same size as one row of words — this allows you to lay it over what you are reading, and move it down the page as you read. This is especially helpful when using a phone book to allow easier reading of numbers. Get help, if you need it, to make this sheet.

» Ensure lighting is bright; using anti-glare light bulbs can assist.

» Prisms may help with double vision; see your optometrist or ophthalmologist

» When possible, ask for text that has been written within the dementia enabling guidelines; for example, if your library produces flyers and you can't read them, refer the flyer producers to these guidelines.[18]

Problem: I spend a long time looking for things and they are right in front of me

Possible strategies:

» The visual cortex is sometimes affected in people with dementia, which means that their brains don't process information coming in from their eyes (which may be functioning fine) properly. This means that it may be harder to recognise common items. Make it easier to see things by reducing visual clutter. For example, leave only essential items on the sink, or on the kitchen bench.

» Label things that you commonly don't recognise.

» Remove clutter, use colour contrasts (e.g. put a white mat

---

18   *http://www.enablingenvironments.com.au/signage*

on your dark bed side table so that you can see your black glasses against this).

» Buy important items in bright colours so that they stand out visually (e.g. bright red glasses, or a yellow phone cover).

Problems when moving around

Problem: I am falling over a lot

Possible strategies:

» Try a walking stick. Many people with dementia find they have visual changes, including things such as changes to spatial awareness and depth perception. For example, stairs that are all the same colour may look like a flat surface, a hole in the floor or a five-metre drop. Using a walking stick gives your brain another message about the height of the ground ahead.

» On stairs, add a contrasting coloured tape to the edge of each step.

» An occupational therapist may do a home assessment and help with more strategies.

» Do exercises that help with your balance such as balancing on one leg or shifting weight in different directions (side to side, forward and back). Some activities, such as dancing or tai chi, are a fun way of doing balance exercises.

Problem: I feel uncoordinated and my body won't always 'work'

Possible strategies:

» Sit down and wait, then try again.

» Use a frame or walking stick.

» Ask for help.

Problem: I'm regularly banging myself when walking through doorways

Possible strategies:

» Add some contrasting colours to the edges of doorways and walls; a lack of spatial awareness or changes to it can make this a regular problem.

» Close the doors, and add signs to them so you easily know which room you want to enter; when you have to open the door to go through it, you become more aware of the doorway.

» Make sure the lighting is bright enough in hallways and keep the lights on in the evening.

Problems related to being with others

Problem: I feel worried and stressed when I know I have to interact with lots of people

Possible strategies:

» Spend time with those people you feel most comfortable with; until our communities become more dementia friendly, it may be too difficult to spend time in large groups of people who either are not dementia aware, or who you are not familiar with

» Be realistic in these situations; real friends will understand that socialising in small groups (two or three couples, maximum) is the most you can easily cope with.

» Avoid joining groups where you are with a lot of strangers, as this may be too challenging to cope with.

» If you want to be a part of larger groups, find a buddy or mentor to support you.

Problem: I can't keep up with conversations, especially in larger groups

Possible strategies:

» Find a buddy to support you in larger groups, if you still want to join them — and why not, we all want to socialise or be part of things!

» Hang out in smaller groups.

» This may also be due to physical hypersensitivity, so let others know you have difficulties with things such as excessive background noise.

» Use reflective listening, which means repeating back what someone said.

» Some people find using ear plugs helpful when they are in crowds, shopping centres or at noisy events.
» At a dinner table or in a restaurant, sit at one end of the table.

Problem: My partner says I am becoming disinhibited or embarrassing
Possible strategies:
» This may be the hardest to control. Try to think before you say anything i.e. try and go over it in your head first and see if it is appropriate before saying it out loud.
» Work out phrases that can qualify what you are about to say, as you know it could be a symptom and what you're saying might not be true.
» Sometimes writing what you want to say, before you say it, helps you see more clearly what you are saying or if someone may misinterpret it; reading it out aloud to yourself first can help as well but of course may not always be possible.
» There may be times you choose not to go out with groups to avoid this happening.
» Care partners can become anxious and embarrassed when this happens, and it is important to find ways to not only work with it, but make sure you know it may happen, and talk about strategies before your dementia progresses. These behaviours are more common in frontotemporal dementia. If you are a care partner or friend of someone this is happening to, think about how it is for them, rather than being embarrassed yourself.

Problem: My friends don't call me anymore and I get lonely
Possible strategies:
» Joining a knitting/fishing/social/other activity-based group can help you find new friends.
» Join a support group in person or online.
» Call your family and friends if you miss them, and tell them.

One lady with dementia told us:

After a while, I decided to just call my closest friends and say I was missing them; after the initial awkward silence, I discovered one in particular (actually, not my 'best' friend) said she felt nervous about contacting me as she did not know if calling in or ringing me would upset me now I've got dementia.

Other problems
Problem: Difficulty swallowing
Possible strategies:
» Change the consistency of your foods, liquidising some if necessary, thickening others.
» Take smaller bites.
» Eat slowly.
» Become aware of the things you have trouble swallowing and avoid these, e.g. meat that is chewy or herbs or leaves with 'frills' such as rocket or coriander may not be as easily swallowed as a piece of iceberg lettuce.
» Seek support from a speech pathologist

Problem: Changes to your sense of hunger or pain, taste and smell
Possible strategies:
» Eat/cook foods with stronger flavours.
» Add more spices.
» Drink stronger coffee or tea; this may mean you need to drink less of it, for health reasons.
» If you are forgetting to eat either because of memory, or you no longer have the sense of feeling hungry or full, use a food diary, or ask someone to remind you; if you don't you will either get very fat or very skinny!
» Be careful with hot taps and boiling water as your ability to know if it is too hot may have changed. You may be able to set or turn down the temperature on your hot

water system to avoid getting burnt; a plumber can also do this for you.

Problem: Your musical or other tastes might change

Possible strategies:

This is not really a major problem, but is quite commonly reported. This happens for some people with dementia and it is only a problem if, for example, family and friends don't know you no longer like ACDC or Mozart, and keep giving you gifts of that type of music, because you 'used to like it', or insist on taking you to restaurants where, in reality, you no longer enjoy the food. Even the style of clothing you want to wear may change.

Tell your family friends if you notice changes like this, as they will find it helpful in supporting you.

Make your home dementia enabling

Some environments are more enabling for people with dementia than others. Environmental design and modification can help people with dementia function better and more easily.

Dementia Enabling Environment Principles were developed by researchers Professor Richard Fleming and Kirsty Bennett from the University of Wollongong. We've included here the principles most relevant for people living at home and have written them from the perspective of the care partner, though people with dementia may be initiating some of these environmental changes. For more information, go to: http://www.enablingenvironments.com.au/adapt-a-home.

Unobtrusively reduce risks: don't make the place feel like a prison because you're trying to keep the person safe. For instance, you could keep the front door open to the outside, but lock the flyscreen. Remove rugs and floor coverings that can be a trip hazard. If you're storing dangerous items in a locked cupboard, then try and do this in an area that the person doesn't access or will be unlikely to notice.

Allow people to see and be seen: this means that the person can easily see key places that they will want to go. For instance, if in the bedroom, you may need a sign to the bathroom if the bathroom can't be seen directly from the bedroom, as well as signs showing how to get to the kitchen and lounge. You could consider changing some opaque doors to glass ones.

Reduce unhelpful stimulation: block out noise, and reduce visual clutter. This may mean avoiding bold patterns on carpet, curtains, wallpaper and tablecloths.

Optimise helpful stimulation: give the person cues about where they are and what they can do there. For instance, placing a seat in the garden encourages someone to stop and sit there.

People with dementia require higher than average light levels. Check lighting in the daytime and evening. Make sure that the lights aren't casting shadows that can be confusing (e.g. the shadow looks like an object or a hole). In the daytime make sure that there is not glare. Also check that reflections from windows and mirrors aren't confusing. Motion sensor lights may be helpful at night.

In the kitchen, make sure that the person can easily find things. Use signs and lists (but not too many!) e.g. label kitchen cupboards with their contents (either signs or a picture). You can even get glass-fronted fridges.

The person may find traditional hot (marked with red and H) and cold (marked with blue and C) taps that you turn easier to use than mixer taps. If you have a mixer tap, add a sign to indicate which direction to lift or twist for hot and cold. Set the maximum temperature on the hot water system so that the person can't be burnt even if they turn on just the hot water.

Make sure that there is good contrast between the floor and the furniture that you want the person to use — it may be difficult to make out a cream sofa on cream carpet in a room with cream walls. If the person has trouble locating the toilet within the bathroom, use a contrasting coloured toilet seat.

Some modern cupboards or doors don't have handles (they are push to open, or have a hidden handle), if the person with dementia is having trouble with these, consider adding a handle.

The environment can also provide prompts for things that the person may like to do. For example, a cupboard with a glass door could hold craft or other activities that the person likes. Or there could be a table in the living room dedicated to these activities.

Support movement and engagement: make sure that there is not too much furniture so that the person has plenty of room to move around.

Create a familiar space: have familiar objects and photos that remind the person who they are. Make sure that furniture looks like its function (no modern chairs that don't look like chairs, or lights that look like space ships). Make sure that furniture is at an appropriate height. Mrs H said:

Signs, including images and descriptions or instructions, were installed in our home as it was becoming far more difficult for my husband with younger onset dementia to remain at home alone due to a reduced ability to plan and remember what things are for or to manage simple instructions without assistance, and this has helped greatly.

Life enhancement strategies and asking for help

Friends, family and others around you greatly impact on how you feel about yourself and perhaps even how you function in the world. Let's say a person with dementia is having trouble managing appointments, her care partner can help by keeping track of the calendar himself, and remind her each day what her appointments are. Or, he may set up an online calendar or organise a paper diary for her and prompt her until she gets into the habit of using it, so that she can continue to manage her own appointments. He may unintentionally make her feel 'stupid' because she can't remember, or help her feel capable of managing her new diary, based on how he offers this support.

It is important for people with dementia to have conversations with those who are supporting them while they still can. If you don't, care partners will try to help in the best way they can, and they might get it wrong. They are human, they love you and want what is best for you, so help them; they are not usually mind readers.

Christine Miserandino, a woman living with the autoimmune condition lupus, in her essay called The Spoon Theory[19] writes:

…the difference in being sick and being healthy is having to make

---

19 *C Miserandino, 'The Spoon Theory', 2003 http://www.butyoudontlooksick.com/ articles/written-by-christine/the-spoon-theory*

choices or to consciously think about things when the rest of the world doesn't have to. The healthy have the luxury of a life without choices, a gift most people take for granted.

She goes on to talk about her feelings with loss of control, and needing to use so much energy to function, saying:

It's hard, the hardest thing I ever had to learn is to slow down, and not do everything. I fight this to this day. I hate feeling left out, having to choose to stay home, or to not get things done that I want to…everything everyone else does comes so easy, but for me it is one hundred little jobs in one.

We recommend you read the whole essay, whether you are the person with dementia, who this chapter is focused on, but also as a care partner, as it gives you excellent insight into the effort required for a person with any disability to function at all.

Be as independent as possible and find ways with your care partner (if you have one) for you to feel in control

Between a person doing something independently, and having someone do it for them, there is a range of support that can be given, and a range of ways of giving the support. Care partners might sometimes do too much for you, but that is because they love you, or because they want to help you. As a person with dementia, it is important in the early stages of your dementia to talk to your care partner about what helps and what doesn't help, and about how you feel. If you don't, how can you reasonably expect them to know what you want, or how you feel.

The invisible disAbilities of dementia mean, for the person diagnosed, it is imperative you talk to your care partner, and family and friends and ask for help. If you don't, help may be given in ways that are unhelpful, or you don't want. As the dementia progresses, you won't be able to communicate as well, so now really is the time. If you are lucky enough to have someone who will be your care partner (i.e. your spouse, partner, child, neighbour or best friend), then involve them, talk to them, and include them. After all, that is what is best for you. And if you have just been diagnosed with dementia and don't have an obvious person to be your care partner, work on setting up services and supports within your community, and with family and friends to support you as much as they are able to.

Help guide your care partner as to the type of support you need; ask for help, talk about these things and make plans together. There may be times for example, when there is an emergency, and they have to take control.

This then means that the care partner gives you the control you still crave; it is difficult for them to know how much is the right amount of support, and some people with dementia will be resistant to help, even when they need it!

Employment and dementia

If you are diagnosed with dementia, and still employed, there is legislation already in place to support anyone living with a disAbility, including people with dementia. People with dementia have rights to remain in paid employment, whilst they are still able to, and may wish to do so. The issue of employment currently is more likely to affect people with younger onset dementia, but as many older people are choosing to work beyond the current retirement age, this may change. See Chapter 8 for more on this.

Driving

Driving is a powerful symbol of competence and independence. It is a routine part of one's adult life. Driving also gives us individual freedom and flexibility. It is difficult to think of giving up the lifestyle choices that come with being able to drive, and it is an issue that causes a lot of stress for people newly diagnosed with dementia and their families. Please see Chapter 8 for more on this.

Chapter 7

SUPPORTING A PERSON WITH DEMENTIA — FOR CARE PARTNERS AND FAMILIES

'Dementia care is caring for people who often do not know they need care, and don't want to be in care; no wonder they may become angry and upset!' (Kate Swaffer, 2008)

This chapter includes information for care partners on looking after themselves, as well as supporting a person with dementia.

Looking after yourself needs to be a priority

As a care partner, active advocate or supporter for someone with dementia, you need to look after yourself so that you're in good physical, emotional and mental condition to continue to support the person with dementia in a positive manner. If you continually put the person with dementia first, and completely ignore your own needs, you may end up getting physically sick or burnt out with exhaustion and then you may no longer be able to look after the person with dementia. If you get too tired and stressed, you may become grumpy and short tempered, and this will affect how you interact with the person with dementia, and therefore the way they respond or react to you.

Emotional contagion is our human tendency to 'catch' the mood of those people around us — so if we spend time with happy people we feel uplifted, similarly, negativity can rub off on us too. People with dementia are more likely to experience emotional contagion than those without dementia. This means that people with dementia are more likely to be influenced by the emotions and mood of people around them. Therefore, when you are stressed, the person with dementia you are supporting will be more likely to be stressed (and this will make your job even harder!). Conversely, if you are calm and more relaxed, the person with dementia is more likely to be calm and relaxed. Ruth Ostrow, who writes for *The Australian* wrote about the Ghandi effect (2016).

When you spend time and energy looking after yourself, you're not being selfish, you're doing what is best for both yourself and the person with dementia. The person with dementia will get the best care from you when you're healthy, happy and relaxed, and you will experience less chance of stress and burnout.

Beware: it is difficult not only to find the time you need to care for yourself as the dementia progresses, it is also very easy to justify putting off finding time for yourself. Often someone will say, 'I'll start that yoga class (or whatever floats your boat to relax and be healthier) next week as I really can't leave X today.' In reality more often than not, next week never comes as far as getting to that yoga class. Getting into the habit of self-care, when the dementia is less advanced or severe will pay huge dividends down the track.

One care partner said, 'I used to never go and do things for myself, but now that I have started to, we are both happier. I felt guilty to start with, but now realise it is best for us both that I do. Apparently, I am a lot less grumpy!'

Being a care partner is often stressful and exhausting

Care partners used to be referred to as the 'hidden patients' because of the impact of caring for someone with dementia. There has been a lot of research and advocacy for care partners, and the stress and burnout that care partners experience is well accepted. In some parts of Australia there are various supports (not often not available in regional or remote communities) and education services for care partners and we encourage you to access these when you need them (see Chapter 5). While much more can be done to support care partners, we are lucky in Australia to have the services we do, especially compared to other countries. Many report, though, that they are hard to find, difficult to access and there simply is not enough support.

When you become a care partner, you may feel like you've lost control of your own life. You may have had personal ambitions, plans and life goals before the diagnosis of dementia. If you are in a relationship you will probably have had many dreams for retirement, or growing old together. Now circumstances have forced you to cut back on those because the person with dementia will ultimately need more of your support, and that takes up your time. Being a care partner will probably mean spending increasing amounts of time looking after that person as the dementia progresses; however we suggest you do not accept the Prescribed Disengagement and start 'doing for' them as soon as they are diagnosed. You can't control how the person with dementia will deteriorate, and you don't know how long you'll need to be doing this job.

It may be worth remembering, the person with dementia does not mean to give you a hard time; they are having a hard time, not only dealing with the various disabilities caused by the symptoms of dementia, but with many other issues such as stigma, isolation and discrimination, and the fear, grief and loss they are feeling.

Your role as a care partner

As a care partner, there are some things you may need to support the person to keep doing themselves, and, eventually, that you may need to do for the person with dementia. It will be helpful to you both if you don't take over all the tasks around the house that were once either shared or done by the person with dementia; support them to continue to be involved in them for as long as possible as if you take them over, or get someone in to do them, you will further disable and disempower the person with dementia. As we mentioned previously when using the swan analogy, if people with dementia stop paddling, they sink, meaning their symptoms can appear to get worse.

Financial and legal affairs of the person with dementia

Always involve the person with dementia in decision-making about their financial and legal affairs. If you have difficulty with the administration of these affairs, get a family member or friend to help. If the affairs are complicated consider paying an accountant, lawyer, or both. Some professionals specialise in this type of work; contacting the Law Society in your state may be helpful to find them. See Chapter 5 about this as well.

Jobs around the house — housework, cooking, gardening and home maintenance

Try to find ways to keep the person with dementia involved in doing these activities. You may need to relax your standards on housework as long as things are hygienic and safe. So you may have to tolerate the house not being as tidy as you'd like or the meals not being as delicious as before, either because the person with dementia can't do the housework as well, or because you don't have time to do things as thoroughly. Some care partners, particularly men, have to learn how to do these household tasks, and get criticised by their spouses with dementia for not doing things properly.

If the person with dementia qualifies for home care services (see Chapter 9 on services) you may choose to use these, or if you can financially afford to do so, you could consider getting paid home cleaning.

Personal care — showers, washing of hair, brushing teeth, cutting fingernails, getting dressed, using the toilet

Try to find life enhancement strategies, which help the person with dementia to do these activities themselves for as long as possible. Sometimes people with dementia don't want to do these tasks when you ask, and forget to do them otherwise. This can be a source of friction for both parties. Try to find ways of persuading the person to do the task through suggestions in the environment (e.g. warm the bathroom, fill the bath and leave clean clothes out), rather than you, the care partner, telling them they HAVE to do it. If they decide not to bathe or shower, it is probably not the end of the world. Having a shower or bath twice a week is enough in terms of hygiene if face, underarms and genitals are cleaned with a cloth on the other days. Sometimes it is not worth the distress it can cause to force the issue.

> *Would you like to know how I sometimes get him to sit on his bed, now that he can no longer understand this function? Sometimes he just freezes and no amount of gentle pushing or leading works. But you know what does? I look up into his eyes and say 'Would you like to dance, darling?' I put my arms up, he automatically assumes the position (we used to do ballroom dancing in our courting days) and then we slowly start to shuffle till I get him to the right spot. It will last less than 30 seconds, but it usually works and I like to think I've given him just a brief flash of a cherished memory.* - From a care partner

Social and medical appointments — keeping track of appointments, making appointments, and providing transport and an escort to appointments

Develop some life enhancement strategies that will work to help the person with dementia manage this for his or herself (see Chapter 6). You may find it helpful to keep a second copy of appointments and act as the Back-Up Brain, and ask for two appointment cards.

Impacts of being a care partner

The impact of being a care partner will be different depending on your relationship with the person with dementia (you may be a spouse or life partner, sibling, child, friend or have some other relationship). It will also differ depending on what your relationship was like before the person got dementia (if you already had a turbulent relationship the diagnosis may make things worse) and your personal circumstances (you may be even more stressed if you have other caring responsibilities, have children in your care, have to work, or have your own health issues). Try not to compare yourself and how 'well you're doing' to other care partners.

About a third of care partners of people with dementia experience clinical depression. One in four care partners of people with dementia have contemplated suicide. Symptoms of depression include:

- feeling sad, depressed or 'blue', or feeling 'empty'
- feelings of hopelessness and helplessness
- feelings of guilt and worthlessness
- insomnia, particularly waking up early in the morning and not being able to go back to sleep
- excessive sleeping
- loss of energy and feeling tired
- irritability and restlessness
- loss of interest in things that were once pleasurable (including sex)
- changes in appetite — not being hungry, or overeating
- difficulty concentrating, remembering details and making decisions.

Positive aspects of caring

Some care partners say that there can be positive aspects to their role, and we hope that you too will find this. Many find that supporting a person they love with dementia allows them to feel positive about themselves later on, knowing they did their best for the person they cared for. It also allows people to make sense of what can be a very distressing time in their life or relationship. The reports below are from research by Peacock et al.[20] Care partners talked about the positive impacts of caring as:

1. Giving them an opportunity to give back — the idea is that they can return the love and care that the person with dementia has given them over their life. Some also describe themselves as role models for their children or others in their family in terms of caring for others.

2. Leading them to personal growth — they have discovered

---

20 *SD Peacock, M Forbes, P Markle-Reid, D Hawranik, L Morgan, B Jansen, D Leipert and SR Henderson, 2010. 'The Positive Aspects of the Caregiving Journey With Dementia: Using a Strengths-Based Perspective to Reveal Opportunities',* Journal of Applied Gerontology, *2010 29(5): 640-659.*

more about themselves, learnt skills for dealing with challenging situations and grown in self-confidence.

3. Discovering inner strengths by connecting with others — they learned to reach out to families and friends for help and support and were heartened by positive responses. They also found strength and comfort from support groups.

4. A sense of competence in the role — many care partners got a sense of satisfaction, accomplishment and competence from being able to provide a safe and loving environment, particularly when there have been challenging situations.

5. Opportunity for a closer relationship and commitment to the care recipient — families spent more time together and became closer in ways that may not have happened without the dementia.

One daughter talked about the honour and joy of caring for her mother:

I feel immensely honoured that I was able to be there for Mum in the last eight years of her life. It created in Mum and me an immensely strong mother and daughter bond. At times I became the mother and Mum was the child, but for most of the time we kept being ourselves and I think that is a really important thing to remember, just be yourself, talk to your mum, do things with you mum, just like you have always done, so long as she seems to be appreciating it.

I kept taking Mum to the opera and orchestra because that's what we've always done together. Even when mum was living in a secure dementia unit, I kept doing this, and eventually it became clear that it was causing Mum distress rather than enjoyment and so we had to stop. Don't ever think your mum can't understand you. Don't ever think your mum can't recognise you. There is so much to learn about communication. Keep talking; keep being familiar and the bond will continue to grow.

A wife talked about the personal growth she experienced:

> *When he suddenly hit a stage of rapid decline to when he went into permanent care were the most challenging, exhausting and at times frightening for me, but strikingly they were also a time of enrichment as I learned new skills in care, and as I became more clearly aware of the fact that I was privileged to have rare moments of finding an activity which made my husband feel useful and important.*

There will be times when you are exhausted, lonely and fearful of your future, and desperately sad about what is happening to the person you are supporting, and therefore, sad about what is happening to you and your relationship with them. Some care partners have said things in frustration like, 'I didn't sign up for this!' and we recommend that, at the times you feel like this, you take some time out for your own needs.

But we promise you, there will be days of sheer joy, exhilaration, love and some incredibly breathtaking moments. You will find your own inner strength; you will get through it. The person you are supporting, even when they can no longer tell you, will love you even more than they did before they had dementia.

Time out for everyone

Regardless of if you are well, and living your life without much stress, the daily grind of living can sometimes get in the way of wellbeing and joy. Let's face it, even simple things like running a home with kids and being a working parent have their days! An older person, who is generally well but may be feeling a few aches and pains or is more tired than they used to be, will have bad days too. We all need time out, at every stage of our life. Days with young children can result in them being placed in time out, or the parent wanting to be sent to their room for some time out! Living with dementia or caring and actively supporting someone with dementia is not much different, except there is a very real need for time out for both of you.

The person with dementia actually needs a break from living with dementia too, even though, of course, they cannot get a real break, as they are living with it constantly. It is not like a broken leg that is getting better. But, sometimes, just being away from their main care partner can give them a break if they are in a place with people they feel comfortable and confident with. It is easy to get lost in the world of dementia, and forget to take a breather, and time away from each other can be helpful for both parties:

Some days, I just need a break from him; he's always telling me what to do, or hovering over me to make sure I'm okay…I know he loves me, but I wish he'd give me more space. Woman with dementia

Try to find ways to have regular time out — small moments every day, and bigger breaks every week. Find an activity that that is of interest to the person with dementia and will occupy them safely, then allow yourself some time (even ten to thirty minutes is enough!) to a have break — read a book, watch television, listen to music, do something you enjoy. The only time you can do this may be when the person with dementia is asleep — you should sometimes prioritise time out for yourself over cleaning the house and doing the paperwork. If you can afford it, get help cleaning the house or with the garden. Some home care packages will offer these as part of the service or you may qualify for carer respite (see Chapter 9).

Get family and friends to visit and take the person with dementia out, or to stay with them while you go out. The person with dementia may enjoy the change in company and scenery. Setting this up with family and friends may also mean you don't need paid carers, who are also strangers to you both, to give you a break later on. Try and set this up as a regular occurrence (e.g. the first Sunday of the month, or every Friday night).

Usually, having a break or finding formal respite options is only something you will do when you feel it is the right time, although, we suggest you are prepared for it rather than waiting for a crisis.

Asking for help

You may not want to ask for help because you want to prove that you can manage, because you don't want to burden others, because you feel it is your responsibility, because you think that no-one else can care for the person like you can, or for many other reasons. It is better for the person with dementia if more people are involved in their life and care. It takes a village to care for a child, and also to care for a person with dementia, so do consider asking for help. You'll probably start with asking for help from close friends and family. Importantly, accept help graciously if offered. If you don't accept help from friends or family member when they offer it they will probably stop offering, as they will feel like you don't want their help. This is also important as they have a life beyond your situation, and the time they offer may be the only time they have available for that week or month.

Ask them to become educated on dementia (for example they could read this book). If you have a few people involved in the care of the person with dementia you (together with the person with dementia if he or she is able to or wants to) may want to prepare some information about the life enhancement strategies and preferences of the person with dementia, to make things easier when he or she is spending time with other care partners.

Even accepting you might need external support can be difficult, as many have said they feel it is 'the beginning of the end'. In fact, accepting services sooner rather than later can mean the difference between everyone living with a better quality of life and the person with dementia being able to stay at home, and you experiencing burnout and no longer being able to continue caring at home.

Interventions for care partners of people with dementia

There have been many studies about what works in supporting care partners of people with dementia. We know that these isolated interventions, such as referring caregivers to support groups, providing self-help materials and offering peer support, do not reduce care partner depression or stress and burnout.

Multi-component interventions do appear to help. These interventions include combinations of care partner education, peer support, case management, individual counselling, exercise or nutritional support. Having a dedicated key worker to work with the person with dementia and their supporters, from the time of diagnosis all the way through the progression of the dementia would be considered optimum support, but is often not available.

Multi-component interventions are more likely to be successful if they:

- provide opportunities within the intervention for the person with dementia, as well as the care partner, to be involved
- encourage care partners to be active participants in education
- offer individualised programs rather than group only sessions
- provide information on an ongoing basis, with specific information about services and coaching regarding their new role
- try to reduce the behavioural symptoms of the person with dementia.

If you can find an intervention with these components in your area, we highly recommend you register. If you can't find the components bundled together, you can try and access some of the individual components separately, for instance go to some education courses, join a support group, and get individual counselling. Alzheimer's Australia is a good place to start for this type of support.

Care partners can be life enhancing for the person with dementia

The relationship between a care partner and the person with dementia is probably the most important in enhancing that person with dementia's life. We humans are social beings; our brains are wired to make sure that we interact cooperatively and with minimal friction with other humans. Hence the way we see ourselves, and the way we function in the world is to a large extent dictated by the way people around us treat us and speak about us.

For example, imagine a rock-climbing student. Their teacher may think that the student has poor coordination and strength (this may be true) and will not be a good rock climber. The teacher doesn't let the student try difficult climbs (he doesn't want her to fail), and takes over in the climbs she does do (rather than letting her figure things out herself). He says 'That's wrong', 'Not like that', 'I've told you that before!' and generally sends the message that he lacks confidence in her ability. The student will probably give up rock climbing after one lesson!

Contrast this with a teacher who recognises the student's coordination and strength limitations, and designs training exercise to build up the student's coordination and strength. He encourages her to try climbs that extend her ability but are not impossible, and encourages her to solve problems, stepping in to support her before she feels too frustrated and making sure that she feels confident and secure in her abilities. He makes suggestions for what she could do differently, rather than telling her that the way she is doing things is wrong.

Since people with dementia often spend large amounts of time with their care partners, the implicit and explicit messages that the care partner sends about the person with dementia's abilities can greatly affect how they see themselves and their mood and self-confidence.

John Sandblom, a person with dementia wrote:[21]

> *We are just changing in ways the rest of you aren't, we have increasing disabilities and the sooner it is looked at that way instead of the stigmas, misunderstandings and complete lies the better for all of us living with dementia. We desperately need others to enable us, not further disable us!*

---

21 J Sandblom, 'ADI2014 What an experience!', 2014 http://www. earlyonsetatypicalalzheimers.com/blog/adi2014-what-an-experience

Chapter 7

It may help care partners to try and understand how the person with dementia feels

In a study in the United Kingdom, in 2015 Damian Murphy asked people with dementia and their care partners to share their feelings and frustrations, and he has given us permission to share his work here. The responses are shown in Table 1. It is illuminating to see how both sides interpret the same situation, since it is relatively rare for people without dementia to really listen to the feelings and frustrations of those living with dementia.

If we listen to people with dementia more (and they are speaking up globally much more), then we may be able to change the focus to living with the disabilities of a dementia, rather than assuming the pseudo death and 'experience of suffering' currently often forced upon them.

There is no right and wrong in the situations presented in Table 1, however, in can be helpful for both care partners and people with dementia to try and understand how the other side is experiencing the same situation. Care partners usually find their role challenging, frustrating and exhausting, but trying to step into the person with dementia's shoes may make the experience easier to understand and respond to. As dementia progresses, the person with dementia may not be able to see things from the care partner's perspective, and it will be increasingly important for the care partner to accept the changes more readily, as well as not blame the person with dementia for the changes.

Stressful and conflict-filled situations arise from a combination of the behaviour and attitudes of the care partner and the changes in the person with dementia. It's not enough to just understand how the other person sees things, though, we also need to think about how to modify our own behaviour so that we are both comfortable in the situation. Both sides could try and modify their responses, but if the care partner has greater ability to have insight and control of their own behaviour, then they may be the one who has to make more changes.

This may seem unfair that the care partner has to make more compromises, but they are the one without the changing cognition and increasing disAbilities. It may therefore be helpful for people without dementia to think about how they would feel if treated and spoken to or about as listed in column 2, to enable them to more positively support a person with dementia.

Table 1: Examples of situations from the perspectives of the care partner and the person with dementia

Care partner perspective	Person with dementia perspective
He doesn't give me any space	I'm quite happy to move away and let her cool off
I'm having to lead a double life here	And that's what annoys me most, you hovering to cover my every mistake, when I don't always make one.
He's not the person he was. He's not the man I married.	I have always loved you, even if I don't remember sometimes. Who is the same person as decades ago?
I try to guide and correct him. I want to make him think and do things for himself	She natters, I feel like the village idiot
'Go and put a sweater on', I said and he came back with his dressing gown on	I go into my room to change as she asked. I know I had to change so I thought it was a good effort. Do I get any credit for that?
She's the cause of all the problems between us. She's got to accept she has dementia	Me the cause? We should all be allowed to forget things
I've had to tell a couple of shop workers about her dementia when she wasn't looking in case she annoyed them	Are you telling people about me? I didn't know that. I don't like the idea of that. You should ask me first. I don't care if you thought it best.
She asks a question but doesn't listen to the answer and asks again	When I ask him something he always says the same thing. It's either 'I've told you already' or 'you don't listen' — so I never actually get an answer'
Sometimes she flies off the handle.	I have to be like that. Otherwise I'm nobody

We've written an alternative way in which the care partner could think about the situation, taking into account how the person with dementia sees things, placed in column 3.

Table 2: Examples of situations from the perspectives of the care partner and the person with dementia, with our added alternative viewpoint

Care partner perspective	Person with dementia perspective	Our suggested alternate care partner viewpoint/ response
He doesn't give me any space	I'm quite happy to move away and let her cool off	If I need space, I could ask for it or plan it rather than blowing up.
I'm having to lead a double life here	And that's what annoys me most, you hovering to cover my every mistake, when I don't always make one.	I could try and give the double life a break sometimes; he doesn't want me watching him for mistakes all the time.
He's not the person he was. He's not the man I married.	I have always loved you, even if I don't remember sometimes. Who is the same person as decades ago?	He loves me, even if he doesn't always remember me. Remember, you have changed as well. Everyone changes.
I try to guide and correct him. I want to make him think and do things for himself	She natters, I feel like the village idiot	I need to back off sometimes, it's better if she feels in control even if she makes a few mistakes. Remember, everyone makes mistakes with or without having dementia.

'Go and put a sweater on,' I said and he came back with his dressing gown on	I go into my room to change as she asked. I know I had to change so I thought it was a good effort. Do I get any credit for that?	I shouldn't sweat the small stuff — she's got a bad memory! It is reasonable to suggest you sometimes change your mind about what to wear too — this may also be a way of reclaiming control
She's the cause of all the problems between us. She's got to accept she has dementia	Me the cause? We should all be allowed to forget things	It is frustrating that she won't accept that she has dementia, but I can't force her. The issue of dementia is causing friction between us; I should just be patient with her memory difficulties.
I've had to tell a couple of shop workers about her dementia when she wasn't looking in case she annoyed them	Are you telling people about me? I didn't know that. I don't like the idea of that. You should ask me first. I don't care if you thought it best.	Next time I will ask her permission before telling people about her dementia. Remember the phrase, 'Nothing about me, without me.'
She asks a question but doesn't listen to the answer and asks again	When I ask him something he always says the same thing. It's either 'I've told you already' or 'you don't listen' — so I never actually get an answer.'	I've got to accept that she will ask the same question over and over — she simply forgets she's asked. If I react negatively it just puts us both in a bad mood. Maybe I can write down information that she asks regularly about in a spot where she will see it.

Sometimes she flies off the handle.	I have to be like that. Otherwise I'm nobody	If I make sure that she feels like an important and valuable person, maybe she won't get angry so quickly. Everyone at least occasionally gets angry. Learning not to sweat the small stuff might be really helpful, as well as accepting the things you cannot change. Remember, it is not their fault they have dementia.

Help them be as independent as possible and to 'feel' in control

Between a person doing something independently, and having someone do it for them, there is a range of support that can be offered, and a range of ways of providing the support. With the absolute best of intentions, care partners sometimes do too much for people with dementia, because they want to help them. The Prescribed Disengagement pathway also tells care partners that this is the right way of behaving.

Let's use the example of giving a short speech at a wedding. The person with dementia may do this independently — writing the speech, rehearsing it, and delivering it. Or the care partner could decide that it will be too difficult for the person with dementia, who may be stressed and embarrassed, and write and deliver the speech — 'Your Mother wanted me to say a few words on her behalf...' Between these two extremes the care partner could help write the speech (delivered by the person with dementia), or read a speech written by the person with dementia.

The way the support is given is key — the person with dementia needs to feel in control, as well as respected and valued. So the person may give the speech, but have little control over it. The care partner could dictate the person with dementia the support he's giving 'I've decided that I'm going to write the speech for you, and I'll help you practise it until you're ready'. Or the person with dementia may not give the speech, but feel control over it — she could enjoy telling the care partner what to put in the speech, and then help him rehearse it until she is happy with his delivery.

Care partners can let themselves be guided by the person with dementia as to the support they need — by offering help, and observing and only stepping in when absolutely necessary. This means that the care partner gives the control of the situation to the person with dementia when possible. It can be very difficult know how much is the right amount of support, and some people with dementia are resistive to help, even when they need it!

Practical help setting up life enhancement strategies

Please read the section on life enhancement strategies, including dementia enabling homes, in Chapter 6. The person with dementia may need your help in identifying strategies that may be useful for them, as well as help with setting up the strategies.

For instance:

- using the computer to putting together lists including pictures, printing and laminating these lists
- helping decide where signs should be put up so that they are obvious
- helping the person learn how to use a new app or other piece of technology
- creating a filing system for notes, photographs and other memories
- checking that the diary and calendar is up-to-date
- filling medication boxes.

Communicating with people with dementia

Most people with dementia will eventually lose the ability to communicate in the same way you communicate, and it can be one of the most frustrating and difficult parts of dementia for everyone. It begins early in the disease process and for many is part of the reason they withdraw. Communication and language is important for a number of reasons. It defines the way others see us, it allows others to communicate with us, it defines the way we view ourselves and it allows us to communicate with others.

There are some common changes in communication abilities for the person with dementia, and everyone will respond and react uniquely to losing these skills. Many have difficulty word finding; conversely, some people may speak fluently, but not make sense. Others may not be able to understand what you are saying, even if they can express themselves. Reading and writing skills often decline, and people may lose the normal social covenants of conversations and either interrupt or ignore someone, or fail to respond completely.

Some may also have a difficulty in expressing their emotions appropriately, for example, feeling and expressing sadness or happiness inappropriately. Some report they pretend to understand, as that is easier than asking people to explain or telling them that they have forgotten, and is also a reason why withdrawing can be common.

Ms P said, 'It is easier to just nod and agree, than embarrass myself.'

Mr S said:

> *When we're out, I can't be bothered joining in conversations cos she always corrects me in front of people, embarrasses me and makes me feel like an idiot. It's easier to just shut up…but then when we get home, she gets angry cos I've not joined in.*

Kate Swaffer's analogy may help explain how to more positively support memory loss or word-finding difficulties, 'For the memory impaired, memory is like a stack of china.' This is why it is important to give people with dementia time to collect what is left of their thoughts, and the time to find the words to tell you about them. Resist the urge to nudge or prompt, or to hurry the person with dementia when finding their thoughts or words, as that will most likely make us stumble and lose our footing — our words — and send the 'plates' crashing down. It you give people with dementia time, it is quite likely they will find their own way to communicate with you.

Find ways to support the person with dementia communicating with you. For example, talking mats is a communication system that uses pictures to help people with dementia make known their feelings and preferences so they can be involved in decisions. There are pictures showing the topic of the discussion (e.g. what do you want to do today), there are pictures showing different activities (e.g. shopping, gardening, socialising), and pictures that the person can use to show how they feel about those activities (positive, undecided or negative). For more information go to http://www.talkingmats.com

According to Mehrabian,[22] communication is made up of three parts:
- 55% is body language
- 38% is the tone and pitch of our voice
- 7% is the words we use.

This explains how others might come across to a person with dementia. Watch your words; they really do matter, and how you say them matters as well. Your tone may impact on how words are interpreted. As comprehension of the words are lost, your tone and body language will impact greatly on the message you are sending. Negative thoughts and moods, negative body language and negative tones will all be picked up by the person with dementia. They may then respond negatively with their behaviour, even if they no longer have the words to tell you they are upset.

Remember to listen to understand, rather than listening to reply. Listening is more than listening to words, especially when the person with dementia may no longer speak well or at all; it includes reading body language as well.

Some ways to help communication with people with dementia include making sure your messages are really clear and concise when you are speaking, defining your message simply, looking directly at the person so they can see your eyes and mouth, using a respectful tone, and being careful of your body language.

---

22 *A Mehrabian*, Silent Messages: Implicit Communication *of* Emotions and Attitudes, *2nd edn, Wadsworth, Belmont, California, 1981*

Make sure the environment you are in is conducive to communication. Background noise, large groups, bright lights and being in new places where the regular routines are not possible, may make communication more difficult. Check that hearing aids are working properly and make sure that glasses are worn when needed. Scottish dementia advocate Agnes Houston talks about 'noise pollution' meaning the background noise in a shopping centre or restaurant, also often found in nursing home activity rooms and general areas, and how it affects people with dementia, disabling them further. Reducing background noise is imperative to good communication with people with dementia.

The person with dementia may no longer have a choice in how they react, but you still do, therefore it is up to people without dementia to change how they communicate. It is up to you to manage your own behaviour and to learn to communicate in a way the person with dementia can understand, and to try and understand them.

Karen Fossum (2003) wrote: 'When your child is no longer a child, you will have to find a new language.' We would not hesitate to consider the communication needs of a child or a person with a speech disability, so it will pay dividends to also to do this for people with dementia.

To better communicate with a person with dementia, reframe your thinking. People living with dementia are not fading away or not all there, they have changed in way that you have not. Let go of what your relationship was, focus on what is possible in the relationship, and what they can still do. People living with dementia are sometimes impulsive. When someone speaks to them with an angry or stressed tone in their voice, they may negatively react to it. You would too; it is no different just because they have dementia.

Communicating 'about' people with disAbilities

When communicating, it is important to use language that focuses on the person's abilities, rather than their deficits (what they can't do), to help maintain positive and meaningful relationships, and to help them retain feelings of self-worth.

If you're communicating about disAbility issues or people with disAbilities including people with dementia here are a few golden rules to consider:

- » Ask yourself if it's necessary to identify the person as having dementia or a disAbility. If you're preparing a document or making a speech at an event or function, you don't label everyone else by their disease or condition, so there is no need to label people with dementia publicly.
- » Always put the person first. When describing someone with a disAbility they are not totally defined by their disAbility, such as in the phrase 'wheelchair bound'. Instead they are a 'person using a wheelchair, or wheelchair user'.
- » Avoid using pitying or sensationalist terms. Most people with disAbilities don't see themselves as 'debilitated' or even 'inspiring' — they just see themselves as people like anyone else.

Language is a powerful tool

Our words do reflect our thoughts and feelings and can show respect or disrespect, and language is a powerful tool.[23] The words we use can strongly influence how others treat or view people with dementia. For example, referring to people with dementia as 'sufferers' or 'victims' implies they are just that, therefore defining them as if that is the sum of their whole experience. This not only strips them of dignity and self-esteem, it reinforces inaccurate stereotypes, heightens the fear and stigma surrounding dementia, and is disabling and disempowering.

Stigma towards people with dementia is still a salient feature of their lived experience and language contributes significantly to this. The stigmatising, negative and disempowering language still being used in the media, and by researchers and clinicians, needs to change in order for the experience of living with dementia to become more enabling and positive.

Until quite recently, people with dementia have had no say in the language of dementia. The language of dementia was generated by health care professionals, people in the media, academics and aged care providers.

---

23 *J Hughes, S Louw and S Sabat (eds),* Dementia: Mind, Meaning, and the Person, *Oxford University Press, 2006*

Now people with dementia are speaking up and saying that some language use in dementia is offensive and unacceptable.

Advocacy organisations such as Alzheimer's Australia, and others around the world, have engaged well with their consumers, to produce documents, which supports a more enabling, positive and respectful communication with and about people with dementia.

One brochure, the 'Talk To Me' guidelines, was developed by the Alzheimer's Australia Dementia Advisory Committee (AADAC), to set out good communication principles when you are talking to people with dementia. The aim was for it to be used to help family, friends, care partners, service providers, health professionals and the general community to better communicate with people with dementia.

Alzheimer's Australia has also produced an updated version of their Dementia Language Guidelines, which they released in 2014, and we recommend that everyone embraces these guidelines, and shares them with family and friends, as well as the health care and service providers sectors. The brochure and guidelines can be downloaded from Alzheimer's Australia's website at fightdementia.org.au/dementia-language-guidelines.

Tips for care partners on supporting people with dementia (from the perspective of a person with dementia)

The following list of tips on how to more positively support a person with dementia is based on Kate Swaffer's 2014 article, '20 Things Not To Do or Say To a Person With Dementia,'[24] and has obviously written from the perspective of a person living with a diagnosis of dementia.

Some of you reading this list may feel criticised or that you've been doing things wrong; that was not Kate's intention when she wrote this list, nor is it ours — we know that you do your very best in looking after your person with dementia. We have written these tips because many people with dementia are unable to communicate these ideas themselves.

---

24 *http://kateswaffer.com/2014/06/05/20-things-not-to-say-or-do-to-a-person-with-dementia*

If the person with dementia themselves could tell you how they feel about the way you 'behave' towards them, you would listen. We hope that when you read this list you'll take it from the perspective of a person with dementia. We hope that by acting on these tips you will improve the lives of people with dementia you interact with, your own experience of caring, and perhaps even your relationship with them.

When we make a mistake or forget:
- » It is unproductive and unkind to keep telling us we are wrong; we may not see things the same way as you do, or we may have forgotten, when you have not. It could even be that we are right and you are wrong; it is statistically impossible for us to be wrong all of the time.
- » It might be better not to argue over trivial things, even if we are wrong; just because you are right doesn't mean that you need to 'correct us'. If you're constantly correcting us, you're disempowering us.
- » It will be supportive not to say, 'But I've just told you that' or 'You've asked me that already.'

- » Try not to say, 'Remember when…' Often we cannot remember, asking us to do something we cannot do can make us feel inferior and causes us deeper distress, which highlights our deficits, and our losses.
- » It may not be helpful to remind us someone has died, if we still think they are alive because we have forgotten they died; there is little point in reminding us and making us sad over and over again, or angry because we may not believe it to be true.

When we change, and keep changing:
- » Don't forget, you are changing too.
- » Meet us in the moment. Stop yearning for us to be the same people we were before the dementia. Grieve the losses and changes as they occur, and then love us as we

are right now. If you don't do this, we feel inadequate and undeserving of your love.

» Changes to our brain are the reason we are changing, and it is not our fault we have dementia. Please don't blame us for the changes — it is hurtful and unhelpful to us both. Many people supporting a person with dementia say they hate the changes and hate being care partners. If we were dying from cancer and not from dementia we would be changing too — would you hate being our care partners in that situation?

» It may feel like you, the care partner is the adult, and the person with dementia is the child (though for some, biologically, the opposite may be true). This doesn't mean that you should treat us like children; please give us the respect you would want yourself, and give other adults.

The words that you use:

» The words you use when talking about us to others are important, they tell us how you see us and feel about us and your role — and many of the words we hear about us, or the tone used, is negative.

» Please use respectful language; many of us don't want to be publicly labelled as sufferers or as demented, many find this disrespectful and offensive. Therefore, please don't refer to us as 'demented', 'demented sufferers', 'dementia victims', 'afflicted', 'fading away', 'disappearing', have a 'dementing illness', an 'empty shell', or 'not all there'.

» Please don't call us 'honey', 'love', 'darling' or anything other than our preferred name, unless we ask you to — this de-individualises us and can feel derogatory.

» It is hurtful if you refer to us as our behaviour e.g. 'aggressives', 'wanderers', 'poor feeders', 'wetters', 'non-communicators' or as 'obstructive', it is negatively labelling us — we are still human beings, we are still mothers, or fathers, or daughters or wives. In our mind, we might still be the surgeon or executive we once were.

When we stop being able to communicate verbally:

» Just because we may not be able to tell you, we can still feel pain; in fact, sometimes when you ask us if we are in pain we may say no when we mean yes, simply because we either may say no to everything as it is easier than admitting we don't understand what you have said, or due to symptoms of dementia such as an acquired dyslexia.

» Please don't assume that because we can't tell you, your words or actions don't hurt our feelings.

» Don't talk over us, or about us, in front of us

» Don't make fun of us directly, or to others in front of us. Many in their interviews also reported this happened often, with partners 'joking sarcastically' about their 'lost capacity' as if it was embarrassing to them, or a joke.

» If we forget how to dress ourselves, or what to do in the bathroom or toilet, please be kind to us and help, but not in a way that demeans or insults us. It is, after all, not our fault we have dementia.

» Don't assume that we don't understand just because we are silent.

We know that you love us and want you to know we love you:
Almost every person with dementia says they never question the love of their care partner; not ever. We know well the depth of love required to be a care partner, and the incredible physical and emotional effort it takes. Sometimes we get angry, we lash out, and we seem ungrateful or resentful, but deep down we know the sacrifices you make to support us, and we know that we need you and your support to live with dementia, and that this will be increasingly demanding as our dementia progresses.

Even when we can no longer tell you, we still love you.

Managing behaviour and mood changes

Empowering and engaging people, in general, requires them to feel valued, involved, appreciated, enabled, trusted, challenged and, importantly, respected. What often happens to people with dementia is from the moment of diagnosis, their doctor will start talking about them to their care partner, rather than talking to them directly anymore. Friends and family often start to do the same. Many people with dementia (and not just in Australia!) have reported this happens for the first time in the diagnosis clinic, and it seems to then continue in other medical and social situations. It is as if, instantly, the person diagnosed with dementia can no longer understand anything at all. This is of course, illogical, but also insulting to the person who is being ignored, and treated as if they are 'no longer there'.

For example, even though a lady with dementia can still speak well for herself, when she and her husband attend a support group, the staff hosting the support group will walk up to her husband and ask, in a whisper, how she is. He regularly says to them, 'For goodness sake, she's just there; why not go and ask her as she can still speak!' Most often they still do not talk to her, even after him saying she can still understand and speak for herself!

It has annoyed this couple to the point they cannot be bothered to attend the support group, as they both feel she is being stigmatised and insulted. This may be an example of what many say they feel is passive stigma within the very sector supporting people with dementia. The person with dementia may have been perceived by the support group staff as being angry, upset and 'non-compliant', but in reality she simply felt insulted and excluded. Her husband may have been perceived as just having a bad day, or that he was stressed in his role as a care partner, which was simply not the case.

One of the most difficult parts of being a care partner is living with the behaviour and mood changes that happen with dementia (see Chapter 3 for a description of these, and why they occur). However, the way that care partners interact with people with dementia can make a great deal of difference in the frequency and severity of these behaviour and mood changes.

Personal care is one area that often makes people with dementia become upset or angry. This may be partly because of the approach that care partners take in reminding the person with dementia to undergo personal care. One older lady with dementia being supported by her husband said:

He wants me to have a shower when it ******* suits him…and I say to myself, he can get lost! He needs to realise it is not all about him and his timetable or plans. I'm still alive so why can't I decide sometimes?

At the end of the day or week, is anyone going to die if someone doesn't have a shower, or even get out of their pyjamas for a day or two? It is also not rocket science to accept that people with dementia will still want to feel like they have some control over their lives and, therefore, it is important, if you are a care partner, to support, and allow that to happen for as long as possible. This may of course, mean changing your own behaviours, attitude or plans. Remember, though, you haven't got dementia, and, in principle, are the one more able to make changes and modify your own behaviour, mood and attitude.

These are broad principles on managing changes, and we encourage readers to seek out further information, support and training. Dr Allen Power's two books[25], *Dementia Beyond Disease*, and *Dementia Beyond Drugs*, will be very useful. Dr Shibley Rahman's two books[26] on living well and living better with dementia will also be extremely helpful. Although written by medical doctors, these books are written in a very 'lay-friendly' way, and easily understood by people without any medical background.

---

1. Think about whether you can live with the mood or behaviour change. For instance, is the mood or behaviour change impacting negatively on the person's quality of life, or their care partners' quality of life? Sometimes people find that

---

25 *GA Power*, Dementia Beyond Disease: Enhancing Well-Being, *Health Professions Press, Baltimore, 2014, Dementia Beyond Drugs: Changing the Culture of Care, Health Professions Press, Baltimore, 2010*

26 *S Rahman*, Living Well with Dementia: The Importance of the Person and the Environment for Wellbeing, *Radcliffe Publishing Ltd, London, 2014,* Living Better with Dementia: Good Practice and Innovation for the Future, *Jessica Kingsley Publishers, London, 2015*

just because a behaviour is unusual doesn't mean the person should be discouraged from it because of society's expectations.

2. Try to figure out the reason/s underlying the mood or behaviour change. — This may be something that has built up cumulatively, something that has occurred recently, or there could be an immediate trigger. Sometimes the reasons don't make logical sense, and sometimes the environment or care partners' behaviour are part of the reasons. If you can't figure out what the reasons are, keeping a diary where you describe the behaviour and the events leading up to it can sometimes help. You will also need to try and be aware of your own behaviour, and how it may be exacerbating the behaviour. Look in the metaphorical mirror. Look at the expectations you are placing on the person with your own tone and emotions, and whether you are feeling burnout, stressed or unhappy yourself. All of these things impact how a person with dementia reacts and responds.

3. Brainstorm a few strategies that may address the causes or triggers for any changes. It can really help to get someone else to help you brainstorm — another care partner or a friend or family member.

For example, if the person seems to be asking the same question over and over because they are worried about being late, then a strategy may be to write a notice on the whiteboard stating the time that you're going to go out, and make sure there is a clock the person can refer to as well. If you can't address the cause or trigger directly, try gently distracting the person. Offer an alternative activity they enjoy doing.

If the person is not distressed or put at risk by the behaviour, but you are upset by it, then think about changing your response, rather than 'fixing' the behaviour. For example, a person with dementia enjoys talking to strangers when she is out, but her care partner thinks it's not appropriate and finds it embarrassing. They fight when he tries to stop her, and he thinks about not taking her out any more. Her care partner could accept her behaviour, and just monitor to make sure that she is not upsetting any strangers or getting in any danger through her conversations.

---

3. Try the strategies and don't give up if the first ones you try don't succeed. Adapt or try different ones, sometimes it takes a few tries to find a solution. Each person is different, and the causes of their behaviour are different.

It can be really helpful to discuss the difficulties you're having with another care partner, or a professional with dementia. For instance, you can call the Alzheimer's Australia's hotline on 1800 100 500.

The Dementia Behaviour Management Advisory Service (DBMAS) is funded by the Australian government to provide support and education on managing behavioural changes in dementia. The role of the DBMAS program is to improve the quality of life of people with dementia and their care partners, where the behaviour of the person with dementia impacts on the support and care of the person with dementia, or the care partner's health. It may be helpful to engage with this service before you resort to medications. DBMAS clinicians will undertake individual assessments and care planning that assists care partners and will also refer you to other appropriate support networks. In Australia you can call DBMAS on 1800 699 799 24 hours a day.

Supporting someone who is experiencing hallucinations or delusions

» Do not argue with the person with dementia, but rather accept the emotions that the person is experiencing.
» Try to validate the person's claims, and then distract them from the hallucination. For example, if the person is afraid of something they believe is present, acknowledge their fear and then suggest moving to somewhere safe.
» Ensure the person with dementia uses aids to alleviate sensory and perceptive challenges. For example, if the person requires reading glasses or hearing aids, make sure they wear them, which can optimise vision and hearing and

may minimise changes in perception. One care partner said, 'When Dad was in the nursing home, one day the staff told me he didn't understand anything. I asked them had they helped him with his hearing aids? Once he could hear, he understood perfectly well!' Sometimes, though, not 'hearing' has nothing to do with the person's auditory abilities, and may be due to the dementia.

» Try altering the environment; ensure areas are well lit and signposted. Reduce noise; adjust the volume on the television, radio and phone so the person can easily hear what is being said.

One lady with dementia said about her hallucinations, 'I've tried to become friends with these strangers that appear, treating them like new friends! It works some of the time.' Her husband said, 'It probably makes us look a bit crazy sometimes, as she talks to them, but it's better than how she used to get frightened and cry.'

Abusive behaviours

Most care partners don't realise that some of their behaviours could meet definitions of psychological or physical abuse. Nearly half the care partners in one study reported significant levels of abusive behaviour towards the person with dementia they care for, and this was more likely if the care partner was depressed or anxious or if the person with dementia had more behavioural and mood changes.

These behaviours could be interpreted as being abusive:

- screaming or shouting at the person with dementia
- using a harsh tone of voice, insulting the person with dementia, swearing at them or calling them names
- threatening to send the person with dementia into a nursing home
- threatening to stop taking care of or abandoning the person with dementia
- threatening to use physical force on the person with dementia

- withholding food from the person with dementia
- hitting or slapping the person with dementia
- shaking the person with dementia
- handling the person with dementia roughly
- speaking unkindly about them in front of them.

If you observe yourself acting in these ways, or feel like acting in these ways, then it will be helpful to take yourself out of the situation, if you can do so safely. Allow yourself to calm down, then get help to manage your stress levels, the situation, your behaviour, or the changes in the person with dementia.

When the person you have been supporting dies

When a person with dementia dies, their family and care partners experience a range of feelings. Grieving for the loss of that person is normal but you may also grieve for the relationship you once had, and the future you expected to have together. Even if dying seemed preferable for the person with dementia due to the level of their disease, you may still feel a huge sense of loss. Guilt may also surface, as you might have had no other choice but to move them into residential care, and that could compound your grief. Some people also find that they have grieved so much during the course of the illness that they feel like they have no feelings left when the person dies, although the feeling of loss and grief may surface later, and quite often unexpectedly.

People have different reactions to emotional experiences. Some reactions to the death of a person with dementia may include:
- shock that someone can die from dementia
- sadness for what could have been, and for what has been lost
- shock and pain
- disbelief and denial
- feeling unable to accept it
- guilt about something in the past
- relief, both for the person with dementia and sometimes for yourself, which can exacerbate feelings of guilt

- anger
- lack of purpose in life now that the caring role has gone —
  many report feeling like there is a 'huge hole' in their lives,
  as they have been so consumed with the role of care partner,
  it feels like there is nothing left to do.

You may experience some or all of these feelings, or others not listed here, and how long you feel them for will vary. There are no rules for grieving; we all react to the grief and loss in our life in our own way. Whatever your reaction to the death, seek support from a grief counsellor if you feel it is affecting your life too much.

Finally, one daughter said, when asked what strategies she had developed to help her manage her role as supporter or care partner:

> It's the strategies that you can't control that are the bother. I was diagnosed with cancer and had a very poor prognosis. The body has its own strategies when given more than it can handle. Once again I emphasise the need for every person diagnosed with dementia to have access to a case worker. Without this, the care partner is left with something too big to hold.

We have been advocating for case workers or key workers for people with dementia and their care partners. They would provide information and support from the point of diagnosis, and through the stages of dementia and decisions that happen as things changes. This person would know your situation and the services that are available in your area. Unfortunately, key workers are currently too often unavailable.

Chapter 8

OTHER IMPORTANT TOPICS

This chapter covers a variety of topics that are relevant to both people with dementia and their care partners. These include driving, pets and commonsense. There are likely many topics we have missed, for which we apologise — feel free to contact us and let us know!

Balancing safety with autonomy

'Safety is what we want for those we love and autonomy is what we want for ourselves.' (Keren Brown Wilson)

People with dementia want autonomy and independence. Families and care partners want them to be safe. This is normal and to be expected.

There are risks in keeping people with dementia physically safe — they are emotional risks for the care partners and families. However, if you keep a person safe against their will you risk many other things and, further in this section, we make some suggestions to enable more activities, including walking outside the home.

There is a real risk that when people with dementia go walking outside the home they may get lost, or they may fall and be injured. However, people with dementia want freedom and a front door key. Families and care partners want the doors locked to know they are safe. People with dementia often feel that this is like being in jail.

One solution is to find ways of enabling the person with dementia to walk outside the house safely, but always talk to the person with dementia about what options they and you feel comfortable with first. We have written this list for people with dementia. If you are a care partner or family member and the person you are supporting with dementia is unable read this themselves, then apply the tips to supporting them, always remembering to talk to them about it, if possible.

Some possible solutions that could enable the person with dementia to keep walking outside the house safely, and stop their care partner or family member from worrying include:

> Put a GPS tracker into your wallet, shoe or keys so that you can easily be located if lost and make sure you have contact information with you (e.g. wallet, wrist band).
> Be willing to walk the same safe route each time, and allow someone to accompany you until you are confident you have learnt the route.
> Take a friend or buddy, or even join a walking group
> Give people on the route you normally use your care partner or a supporter's details.

A man with dementia, when talking about how his son supports him from afar, and only able to visit every 4 to 6 weeks, said:

We also talked about a tracker so that I can keep going out without getting lost and he bought me a fancy watch, which is also a tracking device, for Christmas, which means he can have a look on his laptop to see where I am if I don't answer the phone if he keeps calling. I don't mind at all that he does this, it's a way of stopping him from worrying and it's a really nice watch. Actually it's no different to carrying a mobile phone, is it?

Families may fight about this, and the energy usually put into walking may be spent worrying about it and arguing. Not exercising, especially if you regularly walked for exercise, may affect your emotional as well as physical health, so find ways to keep doing the things you want to do. Find a walking group if you want to keep walking, go to a gym, or ask friend to take you out.

These are some of the negative impacts of not being allowed to walk or engage in activities outside of your home, and the reason why it is so important for you both to find ways to support some autonomy:

- feeling angry, incompetent and that you are being 'restrained'
- feeling like you are 'restrained' from activities such as walking may make you feel disrespected and unvalued
- feeling angry and resentful will cause your relationships to deteriorate
- feeling bored may also impact on your mood or behaviour in other ways, and make your relationships more stressful
- becoming less fit from not exercising will also impact on general mood as well as the person's physical health.

Seeing your symptoms as disAbilities, whilst initially very confronting, will ultimately help you accept support and help. I'm sure many reading this already wear glasses; think of these strategies in the same way, which is why Kate Swaffer started to call them 'life enhancement aids'.

People with dementia often feel like they are in jail, but it is important to be safe, and accept that ultimately some things will need to be done for your safety.

Taking risks

Risk taking is a part of living, and whilst your care partner or family may feel there are times they would prefer you not to take 'reasonable' risks, often there is no reason not to.

One person with dementia said when talking about risk:

One aspect of risk taking behaviour that I think is almost completely ignored is the rational and logical idea that because you are neatly labelled, socially isolated, and have been told, repeatedly, that you are going to die (in general an unpleasant death) that there is little down side to any risky situation. The worst consequence may well be better than the 'better' consequence of not taking that risk.

Residential care facilities are extremely risk adverse, and this has resulted in an overuse of both physical and chemical restraint for people with dementia, which is also a human rights issue. We need to find a balance between not causing undue harm and supporting people with dementia to be allowed to still take some risks, just as everyone else does.

One person with younger onset dementia said, 'I took my pre-teenage kids skydiving, which was 'risky'! What's the difference?!' One older man with quite advanced dementia said, 'Hell, I've got an OBE (over bloody eighty). I really don't care if I get taken out by a bus! In fact, that's better than the alternative!'

It is important for us all to find ways to allow people with dementia to feel like they still have autonomy and control, and in this book we recommend continuing to live your pre-diagnosis life for as long as possible, if that is your wish. That also includes taking risks, so work with your family and care partners to find ways to support your needs and wants in ways that is not too stressful for all of you.

Driving

Driving may seem like an automatic activity, however, it is an extremely complicated task, requiring complex thought processes, manual skills and fast reaction times. Many of the cognitive processes involved in driving may deteriorate early in dementia.

We believe that a diagnosis of dementia means that we are almost certainly unsafe drivers, because dementia, by definition, affects our cognitive ability, and our ability to accurately (and honestly) self-monitor how well we drive.

Some people with dementia recognise that they are not safe drivers and give up driving:

> Due to our brains ceasing to function as it once did, I gave up my licence immediately after my diagnosis. I knew I was a risk and could cause harm to others. With my losing focus and having mental lapses…that's a sure sign that the brain isn't doing its job…I strongly speak out to others with dementia about what they are doing and

tell them they may cause serious injury to others, apart from the possibility of invalid insurance.

Another person with dementia, who eventually gave up his licence, before he was asked to be formally assessed, said:

I feel such a relief that I am not risking someone else's life, and am no longer searching for my car for hours in car parks, or getting lost. I was hiding this from others, including my doctors, and have found not driving has reduced all of the anxiety and stress, as well as my guilt for having kept on driving.

Signs that dementia may be affecting someone's driving abilities

- returning from a habitual drive later than usual
- an increased number of dents and scratches on the car caused by minor accidents, often not with another car but when parking and reversing
- forgetting how to get to and from familiar places
- going out in the car, then getting a taxi or walking home, forgetting you had gone out in the car
- driving down one way roads the wrong direction
- losing the car in places like a familiar car park
- getting lost
- failing to observe traffic signs
- slow reaction times and making slow or poor decisions in traffic
- driving at inappropriate speeds — too slow or too fast
- misjudging speed, distance or turns
- becoming angry, stressed, agitated or confused while driving
- hitting kerbs and gutters
- misjudging car parking
- poor lane control
- confusing the brake and accelerator pedals.

Other factors that may impact safe driving;

» Vision: seeing things coming straight at you and from the sides. Spatial awareness may be affected by dementia. A person with dementia may not see and respond appropriately to traffic signs and signals.

» Acquired dyslexia: not recognising or mixing up the red (STOP) and green (GO) lights, or seeing signs reversed, make it unsafe to drive.

» Hearing: are you able to hear the sound of approaching cars, car horns and sirens, as well as respond appropriately? Do you pay attention to these when in the car? This is especially important for safety on the road for police, fire and ambulance sirens.

» Reading: ability can be impaired. Are you able to read a road map and signs as well as follow detour routes?

» Medications: some medications can affect alertness and impact judgement.

You are legally obligated to report that you have dementia to the licensing authority

It is very important to remember that driving is not a human right. If you are not safe to drive, you may not only endanger yourself but others.

You are required by law to tell your local licensing authority of any medical condition that might affect your ability to drive safely. Dementia, diabetes and some other health conditions all need to be disclosed to the licensing authority due to the fact they may affect driving ability.

The licensing authority in your state will then contact the person with dementia's doctor and ask them to make an initial assessment of the driver's medical fitness. Following this, a formal driving assessment may then be required and, based on the results of these assessments, the licensing authority will decide if the person can continue to drive. Licensing requirements for drivers with dementia, and for assessing fitness to drive, vary across different states and territories in Australia. The cost of assessing fitness to drive is high (can be hundreds of dollars), and is borne entirely by the person with dementia; and there are not sufficient numbers of appropriately trained assessors available to get an assessment.

> *My neurologist, my neuropsychologist, and I all thought I would probably pass a driving assessment. I failed the assessment, with a score as low as 35%, which highlights the fact I had lost insight, and my family also had not picked up it was not safe for me to drive. (Swaffer, 2012)*

If the person with dementia passes the assessment and is able to continue to drive, they will be issued a conditional licence. Conditional licences are valid for a maximum of 12 months after which the driver will need to be reassessed. The licensing board or your doctor will notify you when reassessment is required. Sometimes restrictions are also placed on the licence holder, such as the person can only drive close to home, at certain times, or below certain speed limits.

There can be serious legal consequences if a person with dementia continues to drive and they have not notified their licensing authority, or if they continue to drive after their licence has been cancelled or suspended. If the driver is in a crash they could be charged with driving offences or be prosecuted. Additionally, their insurance company may not provide cover.

Unfortunately, many people with dementia do not recognise that they are not safe to drive. Or if they do, the stress of losing their independence is so high, they lie about their driving ability. Many family care partners also lie about their partner's driving abilities

In one older couple, the husband with dementia said:

> *Our doctor always asks my wife if I am safe to drive…and she always says yes, even though she knows I'm not. She never learnt to drive you see, so what would we do if I can't drive anymore?*

Doctors are also loath to confront the issue, for a number of reasons, not least because it may prevent the person from attending to other health needs. Doctors are often overly protective of patients with cognitive disabilities or dementia, and are reported to say they do not wish to take away a person's independence or damage their relationship with the person.

Discussing stopping driving

Driving is frequently an issue of contention between people with dementia and their family or doctor. One husband said:

> *I don't know how to bring up the topic of my wife's driving, and her possible dementia. I feel she most likely has dementia, and I am pretty sure she is unsafe to be driving, and I have asked her doctor to assess her for both, but he says there is no need. What happens then, if she kills someone on the road? Is it the fault of her doctor, or the system, and I wonder, will our insurance policy still be valid, especially as I have formally raised my concerns with her doctor?'*

Driving is not a human right; driving is a privilege. This is one of the few issues that we strongly advocate discussing with your doctor, care partner and your family. Also, if you are a person diagnosed who is reading this, we ask that you read this section with an open mind. We realise that we're saying things that you don't really want to hear. The risks involved in a person with dementia continuing to drive with being assessed for driving safety, probably outweigh the risks to independence and self-esteem of actually losing your licence.

A few points for care partners and families to consider

Actions such as hiding car keys or licence or disabling the car could seem very disrespectful and hostile. Trying to take away the person's freedom without their permission is very likely to lose you respect and trust, may cause great anger towards you and even jeopardise your relationship. These actions also may not be helpful in reducing the risk of driving, as the person may continue to drive without a licence, have their car re-abled, or simply go out and buy a new one if they have the funds to do so. It is best if you can get the person to agree to stop driving when you truly believe they are no longer safe to drive, or to talk to their doctor about it (even, sometimes, if they are reluctant and unhappy about this decision).

The University of Wollongong has published a freely available booklet 'Driving and Dementia — a Decision Aid'. You can visit the University of Wollongong's website at smah.uow.edu.au/nursing/adhere/drivingdementia to download the guide.

You may need to address the issue of driving with a person with dementia

We suggest families and care partners start discussions as early as possible after a person's diagnosis. Don't choose a time when either their driving has become questionable (such as just after a driving incident or crash), or at some other time when either of you is stressed or agitated.

» Have short and frequent conversations, rather than one long discussion.

» Concentrate on the person's strengths and remaining abilities, and the positive aspects of other options.

» Acknowledge that giving up driving is difficult emotionally and affects their independence and sense of status.

» It might be helpful to focus on the nature of the disease, for example, safe past driving records have no bearing on their safety (or the safety of others) as a driver with dementia in the future.

» Be respectful and try to understand how the person with dementia will be feeling.

» Consider what driving means to the person. Owning and driving a car or other vehicle can mean more than just mobility and independence to a driver. It can be a sign of status, a hobby and even a job.

» Remember, they have already lost many 'things' due to dementia, and will continue to lose memories, capacity and function — having their drivers licence taken away adds to the difficulty of accepting all of the other losses.

» Offer alternatives to driving (see section below).

It is important to have these conversations, though, as being forced to sit a practical driving test, and failing, can be very traumatic.

My GP suggested I think about giving up driving before I was forced to...I soooooo wish I had taken this advice, as failing my driving test was excruciatingly painful. I cried for days, and then felt really angry. (Person with younger onset dementia)

You can also contact the local licensing authority to discuss your concerns. The licensing authority may contact the driver and advise that a medical and driving test is necessary. The emotional and physical toll of having a driver's licence revoked can include:

- significant loss and grief — it feels like a death and it may even feel worse than receiving the diagnosis of dementia
- loss of independence
- loss of control
- loss of privacy
- lower self-esteem and self-worth, feelings of incompetence
- perceived loss of social equality from not having a driver's licence
- it may affect employment
- increased isolation and loneliness
- increased guilt, stigma, sense of being a burden, which then increases the sadness
- tension and anxiety relying on others
- reduced family income; loss of work hours for partner to provide transport
- buses and taxis can be too difficult for people with dementia to negotiate
- sense of wellbeing significantly impaired

Alternatives to driving

When people stop driving they often stop making social trips, like visiting friends, family, attending functions or participating in hobbies. It is important that social contacts are maintained to try to reduce the isolation that many with dementia will be experiencing. One person with dementia said, 'It felt a bit like a death, and in a way was like that. My friends were supportive in the beginning, then just got back on with their lives.'

People with dementia can be helped to reduce the need to drive and to find alternatives for getting around, for example

» When a person can no longer drive due to a health issue (including dementia), their doctor can complete the documentation to gain them access to the Assisted Transport Subsidy Scheme (ATSS), which gives the person a discount using taxis. However, these vouchers cannot be used with services like Smart Car, as they are considered to be hire vehicles, rather than taxis. If the person you are supporting has lost their drivers licence, and are able to manage using taxis, it is helpful to find a service where you can get the same driver. The rationale for this is that having someone the person is familiar with will reduce anxiety, and with their permission, you can also give the driver your contact details, in case the person appears to be unwell or is having trouble remembering where they are going. It is very supportive and helpful to have a familiar driver.

» Offer to support the person by driving them (or ask other family members of friends to drive them) to appointments, social gatherings and to go shopping and to access services.

» Encourage the use of buses, trains or taxis when possible, although this can be difficult to navigate for many with dementia.

» Encourage walking, when possible. The use of GPS technology can help if someone starts to get lost. For those people with dementia who have a phone with access to the internet, there are very useful maps and other apps available.

» Provide a wallet or purse sized care pack with emergency contact details, as well as the person's name and home address. This can assist if there is an accident or some other incident occurs and the person with dementia is unable to tell someone.

» Look into community transport services available in your area (see Chapter 9 on services).

» Encourage the use of home delivery services for food, medical prescriptions and the local library.

Employment and dementia

People with dementia and care partners of people with dementia have rights when it comes to employment, but it is worth noting up front, so do employers. This section details as much as possible what they are, but please note, it is not legal advice for either the employer or an employee with dementia, however well informed. For anyone who wants to remain at their place of employment, we would suggest you seek rehabilitation counselling or other advice, and for all workplace relations and legal advice you should always seek legal advice.

For some people diagnosed with dementia, leaving work, if they are employed, will be their most preferred option. Doing things like spending more time with family and friends, or hobbies, or getting on with their bucket list will become their priority. But many people diagnosed with a dementia, particularly younger people, want to continue to work and live a productive and meaningful life. There are many self-advocates for dementia speaking up about how they want to keep living and working. Many could, and perhaps should, have remained in paid employment, but currently the system does not support or even encourage them to do so.

Prescribed Disengagement may be the main culprit behind most people with dementia quitting work. The health and social sectors do not support employment, or even suggest it is possible to remain employed, after a diagnosis. Within the workplace, stigma and discrimination is still prevalent, and this also is a reason why people with dementia are not supported to stay at work.

Whilst people with dementia still have capacity and abilities, every effort must be made to support them with reasonable adjustments to allow them to continue working for as long as they may wish to remain employed. I some cases, even where an employer provides a 'reasonable adjustment' the person with dementia may not be able to remain employed.

Continuing to work as a care partner

Care partners of people with dementia have rights to be supported in their continued employment. Unpaid caring responsibilities may demand a lot of time and affect people's capacity to participate in the workforce. The Australian Human Rights Commission (2013) has a toolkit for supporting carers in the workplace, and we would recommend you access it from the resource list in this book.

Care partners may wish to remain in paid employment too, but if you take on the role of full-time care partner, there will likely come a time when you will no longer be able to work. For younger people who have a partner with younger onset dementia, this may not be the best option, as, if they go into residential care or when they die, you may well wish to work again, and gaining employment may be more difficult after a period of unemployment. Sometimes finding ways to support the person with dementia so that you can still work some of the time is a healthier option for you both.

There are minimum legal requirements as to the support that should be provided for people with caring responsibilities in the workplace. These include provisions under the National Employment Standards (NES). Employment laws to support carers in the workplace prescribe the following as a minimum under the NES:

> » Requests for flexible working arrangements — available
> to parents or carers of a child under school age or a child
> under 18 years with disability.
> » Parental leave and related entitlements — up to 12 months'
> unpaid leave, plus a right to request an additional 12
> months' unpaid leave for the birth or adoption of a child.
> » Personal/carer's leave and compassionate leave — ten days
> paid personal/carer's leave and two days' unpaid carer's leave
> per occasion. In addition, two days' compassionate leave
> per occasion is also available if a member of the immediate
> family or the household has sustained a life-threatening
> illness or injury. (Australian Human Rights Commission,
> 2013, *Supporting Carers in the Workplace: A Toolkit*)

You can find more information on the NES from the Fair Work Ombudsman at www.fairwork.gov.au.

People with dementia and employment

This advice is written from the Australian perspective, and we would always suggest you seek legal consultation for your own situation and in case legislation has changed since the time of writing.

As an employee with dementia, if you have capacity, and are capable of fulfilling your current role, or can do so with reasonable adjustments and want to remain in paid employment, you have a right to remain employed.

As an employer, the important point to remember is it is a person's legal right to remain employed and to expect support to 'reasonable adjustments', providing this does not include adjustments that would impose an unjustifiable hardship on the employer (in the case of adjustments to enable a person to perform the inherent requirements of a job), or which would be unreasonable.

There will be circumstances where the employer might say that the person with dementia is unable to meet the requirements of the job even with reasonable adjustments. It is therefore important to acknowledge that in some cases even with 'reasonable adjustments' a person with dementia may not be able to remain employed.

Any person who has a disAbility, mental health or medical condition (including dementia) which impacts on their work is eligible for disability services such as auxiliary aids, meaning equipment (other than a palliative or therapeutic device) that provides assistance to a person with a disAbility to alleviate the effect of the disAbility (*Disability Discrimination Act 1992*).

A person's disAbility may require supporting documentation from the employee's treating practitioner (e.g. doctor, neurologist, psychologist, psychiatrist) to determine eligibility, but support for disabilities cannot legally be denied. The *Disability Discrimination Act* says: 'It is unlawful for an employer or a person acting or purporting to act on behalf of an employer to discriminate against a person on the ground of the other person's disAbility or a disAbility of any of that other person's associates...'

It is not discrimination under the *Disability Discrimination Act* to:

- fail or refuse to employ a person for a job, or fail or refuse to transfer or promote the person to a job
- terminate a person's employment in a job, but, this is only if:
- the person is unable, or would be unable, to perform the inherent requirements of that job; and this inability cannot be remedied by making a reasonable adjustment.

If it is possible, with the appropriate support for disAbilities, for a person with dementia to remain employed, there are benefits not only to the individuals, but their families, the health care sector and society as a whole. It also supports the reduction of stigma, discrimination, isolation and reduces the misperceptions others have about dementia.

The *World Alzheimer's Report 2015* discussed the rights of people with dementia to be and remain employed, and actively and publicly encouraged employers to consider employing people with dementia. People with dementia are being employed in dementia-friendly communities initiatives and campaigns, in the same way that indigenous or gay people are employed for Indigenous- or gay-friendly projects.

Supporting disAbilities in the workplace

It is important to remember that many of the disAbilities of a person with dementia can, and should, be supported in the same way they are for any other disAbled person. These may include support for learning or other cognitive disAbilities, as well as visual, hearing, mobility or other physical disAbilities. The following is a list of disAbilities, followed by a list of strategies and resources. Both lists may not cover every disAbility or possible support. Research shows there is a much higher chance of successfully supporting a person with dementia to remain employed and to successfully use assisted technology or other supports if introduced to them at an earlier stage of dementia.

The following is a list of some disAbilities caused by the symptoms of cognitive impairment or dementia, which can be well supported to maintain some level of functioning:

- dyslexia

- word finding or understanding, or changes in comprehension abilities vision impairment
- spatial or other sight impairment affecting mobility
- hearing impairment
- learning difficulties
- memory impairment, e.g. retention of new information
- motivation may be lower
- organisation and planning abilities may have changed
- reduced attention span, difficulty starting or maintaining activities
- judgement and reasoning changes
- loss of insight and some social skills.

Strategies to support the disAbilities of cognitive impairment and dementia in the workplace (and in life)

Strategies to support the disAbilities of cognitive impairment or dementia can include Assisted Technology (AT). AT is any product or piece of equipment used to maintain or improve the functional capabilities of people with disAbilities and can benefit employees who are experiencing disAbilities of dementia. The following is a list of AT, support software and other strategies, although not exhaustive, as new AT is being developed all the time:

» Support for acquired dyslexia. This may include simple things like additional software for spelling, or providing the minutes of meetings as a Word document, as well as having them recorded.

» Time management support. This includes things like using electronic reminders and calendars when online. Purchasing a time management program may also be helpful.

» Using email or notes to record meeting. If you have a conversation, it might assist the person with dementia to follow it up with a précis of what has been discussed or requested; if it is via email, then you both automatically have a record of the conversation.

Up-to-date computer with USB ports on the front to allow easy plug-in of headphones and other equipment.

» Large-screen LCD monitor that is easily adjustable on a swing arm so that it can be positioned to suit a range of users.

» A4 scanner allowing hard copy material to be converted into electronic text, so that it can be used with specialised software and enlarged or read from the screen.

» A3/A4 printer allowing material to be easily printed in enlarged text.

» Dragon NaturallySpeaking speech recognition software. This software provides users with the ability to write essays and emails and even explore the web by voice command. It can be very useful for students who have difficulty working at a keyboard or using text.

» Zoomtext software provides text magnification along with screen reading so that users can listen to the material that appears on the screen. This product is designed especially for people with vision impairment

» Read & Write software is designed for use by people who have a learning disAbility. It provides features such as enhanced spelling and grammar checking, word prediction and screen reading in an easy to use package.

» Spectronics is an inclusive learning technology designed by an occupational therapist, applying technology options to assist people with cerebral palsy and spinal cord injury to achieve their goals, and works well for some people with cognitive disabilities and dyslexia.

» Word finding or understanding, or changes in comprehension abilities can be supported with the use of visual aids, and alternatives such as audio or video files.

» Vision impairment can be supported with computer software for screen enlargement; audio aids may also assist.

» Spatial or other sight impairment affecting mobility can be supported following enabling environment design principles.

» Hearing impairments can be supported with visual aids and

hearing aids, e.g. using microphones for speakers during meetings.

» Learning and/or memory impairment can be supported with electronic reminders or having a support person at work to act as a mentor and buddy.

» Additional time may be required to complete tasks.

Prior to and during work meetings:

» Staff with dementia may need to be able to comment or ask questions as they think of them, rather than be asked to wait, as they may not always be able to 'hold that thought'.

» Provide meeting minutes in a verbal format, e.g. podcast or a simple set of spoken minutes.

» Provide reading material in advance of meetings.

» All meeting papers should be sent as early as possible.

» Papers should be presented in a clear, organised and numbered manner in the folder.

» Provide and allow the use of an App called SoundNote so employees can record meetings for future reference whilst typing their own notes. This app then allows you to go back to the recording and fill in missing notes, as well as having an option to email notes to others.

» Feedback can be provided from members in writing prior to the meeting if they wish to do so. This feedback can then either be distributed to other members for consideration prior to the meeting or presented at the meeting by the member, another member or chair.

Natural supports can easily be provided; support in a workplace could mean assistance through relationships, buddies or mentors, as well as interactions that allow the person with dementia to work in a job of their choice in ways similar to any other employee needing support.

It is important to remember the language you use can be inclusive and respectful, or it can be exclusive, demeaning and disrespectful. Make sure all staff read the recently updated *Alzheimer's Australia Dementia*

Language Guidelines 2014. Refer also to the section on dementia enabling environments on page 134.

Respect and communication in the workplace

Respect, kindness, patience, common sense, and using good communication skills are simple steps to support a person living with the disAbilities of dementia. Learning to communicate with a person with language or cognitive impairment is as important as learning to communicate with someone who has lost their speech after a stroke or some other disAbling condition. It is not the person's fault, and it is up to others without disAbilities to make the time and effort to learn about the disease, and how to best communicate.

We are hopeful that in the future, employers, and ultimately legislation, will also support any time off during the diagnostic process with sick leave in the same way you would if the person had been diagnosed with another terminal illness such as cancer. It should not be a reason to have to resign.

Organisations, services and legislation supporting disAbilities in Australia

- Employee Assistance Program
- Australian Human Rights Commission
- Australian Human Rights Commission — Mental Health in the Workplace
- Blind Welfare Association
- Guide Dogs Australia
- Royal Society for the Blind
- Health Insite
- Disability Information and Resource Centre Inc (DIRC)
- Deaf CanDo
- *Australian Human Rights Commission Act 1986*
- *Disability Discrimination Act 1992*
- *Age Discrimination Act 2004*
- *Racial Discrimination Act 1975*
- *Sex Discrimination Act 1984*

Travelling and dementia

When you have dementia travelling can be less enjoyable as it changes the experience of travel from holiday mode and relaxation, to one of increasing levels of hard work, and possible anxiety and stress for the person with dementia (and their travelling companions, if they have them).

Travelling can be tiring, difficult and stressful for anyone, with or without health issues — there is lots of new information (new locations, new accommodation, different food, possibly different language) to process, the days can be long and there are different time zones to cope with. The brainpower available is used up just in managing the essentials of travelling, the 'paddling' underwater becomes much harder and there is not much energy left for anything else (such as having fun!). For people with dementia with symptoms such as reduced spatial awareness and depth perception and acquired dyslexia, things like understanding signs and traffic lights can be worse than when at home, in part due to the crowds, noise and fatigue.

If you enjoy travelling, then you may want to continue doing so. You may also have places on your bucket list that you still want to visit. You may need to travel to see family, or visit friends. You may need to travel for medical appointments, or because of work.

When travelling, it is possible that you will discover a few new things about living with dementia that may not be so evident when you are at home in your regular routines. If your way of coping is denial, the denial bubble may not work when you are experiencing more difficulties. Travel can highlight the deterioration or progression of dementia, which can be quite confronting for the person diagnosed and whoever they are travelling with.

Kate Swaffer wrote this after a trip to New York:

> *It is a major juggling act for us both, every waking hour. Don't get me wrong, we are having a good time, but the strain of travelling with Mr Dementia is showing on both of us. My darling husband has made every effort to make sure we do things together, and even spoilt me with a helicopter ride yesterday, something I'd not done before, and was lucky enough to sit in the cockpit with the pilot.*

But below the surface, or hiding behind our seemingly happy holiday snapshots, is a lot of very strained paddling by me, and a large amount of juggling by both of us to manage being on holidays without things like me getting lost or run over. It is extremely tiring and stressful for Pete.

Her husband Peter said during that same trip, 'I can now see how much you must struggle at home while I'm at work all day.'

Should you travel at all?

As a care partner, the person's level of dementia, and mood and behaviour will probably dictate your travel plans (where to, for how long), or if you travel at all. A short one night or weekend break, a visit to friends or relatives, or a longer trip away on holiday might all have to be thought about. Do your homework first and be as prepared as possible, before you depart.

Paul in the UK, whose wife is advancing with her dementia said:

I have now come to the conclusion that it would be ridiculous to expect Maureen to travel. Travelling will only cause distress: Maureen is hardly familiar with our home. Taking her out of it would be a silly thing to do. She would not know where she was: how could she? When we returned home she would be confused again and take time to settle. It is my role is to seek to minimise distress. Travelling will only increase it. Maureen's world is shrinking she is struggling to cope with where we are now. Taking her away from her familiar surroundings would be ridiculous and reckless!

This is not something I wanted to accept. I need to travel to see people and nice places. Maureen will no longer be able to accompany me. She will feel deserted and frightened if I leave her. In my hour of need, and there have been many, she never left my side. I told her the other day it is 'until death do us part', and it will be. I will stay by her side.

Planning for your trip

Make sure you have copies of all of your travel arrangements. If you no longer drive then you will need either a passport or an Identification card as some hotels will not accept you without photo ID. You can get an ID card that has your photo, usually from the transport authority in your state or territory or your post office.

If you can book out of season this will mean there are less crowds to cope with and the staff, or your hosts, will also be more relaxed and maybe able to give you more time and support to ensure you have a good holiday.

If you are travelling with someone with dementia, it is a big help to take others on the trip with you — another person can help find your way, make decisions, stay with the person with dementia (for instance if you need to go to the toilet) and help with the luggage. Having others along with you can also be fun, provide more company, allows you to get time to yourself and can take over if you get sick.

If you'll be visiting friends or family, ensure they have some understanding not only of dementia, but the type of dementia you have, as well as the level of your disabilities and the support you might need. Being informed, prior to your arrival, can minimise stress for everyone. Let them know about routines, possible triggers (things which may cause distress), diet and any other thing that might help to support the person with dementia. If you have to take medication at specific times and this is related to when meals are taken or as part of a bedtime routine, knowing this will help the host.

Transport

If you're flying to your destination, it is worth noting that some airlines are working towards being 'dementia friendly' as are some other public transport organisations, although it's probably best to assume there won't be any support, which might cause added stress to travelling. Limitations on mobility, dietary needs or other support may need to be accounted for in advance.

You can reasonably expect support for disAbilities, including having someone take you to the luggage carousel, or to the next leg of your flight. All you will need to do is phone the airline you are using to ask for this service, as most now provide this support.

If you're travelling by public transport, think how you will navigate this on your own, and how you will cope with noise and crowds? What will you do if your journey is delayed or you get lost?

Accommodation

When booking a hotel, you may want to ask for a quiet room. Sometimes rooms at the ends of corridors, or away from the main parts of the hotel, such as restaurants, may be quieter.

Book into a room for people with disabilities, especially if you are still managing well enough to sometimes travel alone. In a better hotel or motel these rooms are usually on the ground floor, and they also have emergency cords in the bedrooms and bathrooms; very useful if something happens and you feel too stressed to leave the room. Asking for this kind of help can be hard to do and you may have to give up some pride to do so.

Many hotels and motels are now dog friendly, so call ahead to ask if you wish to travel with your dog. In the United States and Canada most properties in the Hilton hotel chain allow dogs on site, as does the Hilton hotel in Adelaide.

Things to pack

Take enough medication for the trip plus two days, and a signed letter from your doctor with a list of what's prescribed if travelling overseas, and the details, in case you need to talk to a doctor or pharmacist while you are away. Take this in your hand luggage if you're flying, and take copies of the letter from the doctor.

- » Put together a medical profile including allergies, as well as general likes and dislikes and dietary choices in case of emergency hospital admission
- » Take copies of reading glass prescriptions and any other similar medical records
- » Make sure you have plenty of personal items, as sometimes needing to purchase a different brand could be stressful
- » Laminate a sheet to take with you, listing all the things you need to pack — you may have someone help you when you are packing to leave but be packing on your own to come

home or between destinations. A help sheet is very useful as you may well be tired from travelling and having trouble remembering or functioning as well.

Travel insurance

We've found a couple of travel insurance companies that do not exclude dementia if it is a pre-existing condition, but you will need to search at the time you intend to travel, as these change often. We recommend you double-check with your insurance provider that both you are (both) fully covered.

Other considerations

» It could be helpful to let your doctor know where you are going and make sure you have details of a local doctor and an out-of-hours practice; communication between both doctors will be helped by doing this.

» If possible, scope out your destination beforehand. Will there be stairs? Is there an escalator or a lift? What about the environment? The flooring and carpets? Are there any hazards you need to look out for? These could include loose rugs, wires, access to different areas, and so on.

» Ensure your hosts have contact details for one of your friends or other family in case you are taken ill and someone is needed to care for your relative or to come to fetch either of you, and that your family at home have full details of your itinerary.

» Take lots of photos and videos; if possible, get a camera that dates and names locations you took them as remembering where you took them could be difficult.

The value of pets

Research tells us that people who have pets have better mental and physical health. Dogs in particular seem to have positive effects for people. Here are some reasons why pet ownership may be healthy for us:

• pets provide companionship, give unconditional love, make

us feel less isolated, and give us someone to talk to who never argues back

- stroking and interacting with a pet can make you feel calmer and less stressed
- taking a dog for a walk will make sure you get some exercise
- having a pet gives you a reason to get out of bed, and structure and routine to the day
- being a pet owner is an important social role, and being able to care for an animal may be an important part of someone's self-image.

Companion dogs are now being trained to support people with dementia allowing them to remain more active and independent in their community. People with dementia receive support in working with their companion dog.

A consumer directed care package will help care for a pet if a case is made that the pet makes an important contribution to the person's wellbeing. For example, if the person with dementia needs help walking the dog, this may be organised as part of the package. Some nursing homes will let residents bring their pets with them, others may have visiting pets as therapy (usually dogs).

Common sense in dementia care

Common sense is often missing these days, not just in dementia care, and the need for everything to be strictly evidence based is prevalent in the health sector. However, it is extremely logical that commonsense, alongside evidence, should be introduced into dementia and aged care, especially residential care, where we heard stories of people who had not been outside since moving in.

The desire and intent to improve and to provide better care for people with dementia seems high in the sector, especially amongst service providers and researchers, although, it seems there is a long way still to go until best practice is the norm, rather than the exception.

Whilst we do need evidence-based practice, we also need some good old-fashioned commonsense in dementia care plans. The sector has a high level of education and evidence-based research to inform practice and the suggestions in this section combine both evidence and common sense.

We all know the positive effects of sunlight on mood, and the health issues associated with vitamin D deficiency, and then we wonder why people living in residential care become unhappy and their dementia symptoms get worse. Surely it is logical that never going outside into the sunshine will lower mood and happiness and reduce the vitamin D in our bodies, both potentially negatively affecting dementia symptoms.

We all know the positive effects of daily exercise, but most people in residential aged care are lucky to get any exercise at all, other than to the bathroom or dining room, and that is often with help, to save time. We know the negative effect on our physical and emotional health when we don't exercise, including falls risk, and this also applies to people with dementia.

We all know the positive effects of healthy, nourishing food made from fresh produce, which is served to us in a way that looks appetising and appealing, and smells and tastes good. We also know that we would not want to eat food that was boring, mushy or that we dislike. This is a common experience for people with dementia.

We all like to feel we have control and having some control of our own life increases our positive outlook and self-esteem. And yet, all control is taken away from people living in residential care. This is in spite of the fact residential aged care is beautifully marketed as your new home. Really? Your new home but you can't get out (no, you are not given a key), and you have almost no say in how you live, when and what you eat, the music you listen to, or the activities available to you?

People with dementia are already losing control of their functioning, their capacity, their abilities, so to take even more control away from them when they go into residential care can only make them sad, unhappy, anxious and even angry. This loss of control might also have something to do with the 'behaviours of concern' many are currently being physically or chemically restrained for.

We all know the positive effects of meaningful activities, of engaging in the hobbies and activities we enjoy, such as gardening and music. Yet,

I often see activity rooms in residential care and day respite full of people looking bored, playing Bingo or doing other meaningless group activities. This allows for fewer staff, and less work in planning, but is not person-centred in any way.

We all know the positive effects of normal socialising and going out to community events, yet rarely do people in residential care get taken out to social or community events like concerts. Instead, we bring these things in-house to the residents, all sitting around the day or activity room. It would almost certainly be far more fun going OUT to the theatre or the movies, and not doing so, negatively affects people with dementia.

We know that many family and friends drop away when someone is diagnosed with dementia, and then, when they move into residential care, visitors dwindle even more. Research clearly supports this. So, supporting people who live in a residential care homes to socialise in normal ways, has to be good for them. Improving mood, happiness and wellbeing, perceived or otherwise, as well as giving back some sense of control has to be the right and sensible thing to do.

We know that for other diseases or illnesses, lifestyle changes improve our chances of recovery or reduce the impact of the illness. Increasing exercise, rehabilitation, improving nutrition, getting sunlight and working our brains hard are all positive interventions that improve our wellbeing, even if they are not a cure.

It makes good common sense to provide care for people with dementia that provides the same support as any other disease. Who knows, if they start to feel happier simply due to increased serotonin from exercising, and have less falls because of some regular resistance and balance exercises, it might actually be good for them, even slow down the deterioration caused by dementia. It might reduce 'challenging behaviours' as well.

If you are supporting a person with dementia, whether you are a family care partner assisting someone living at home, or working in a residential care facility, think about how common sense would benefit their wellbeing. The benefits far outweigh the disadvantages and, mostly, it will cost very little to implement some very simple changes, that will reap significant rewards for people with dementia and those supporting and caring for them.

Celebrations

Celebrations such as Christmas or family weddings are often a very stressful time anyway, and even more so for people with dementia and their families. With the added commitment and time required of being a care partner, simple things like the shopping, cooking, gift purchasing and cards can be more time-consuming and arduous than for many others. The financial constraint dementia places on many individuals and families can also impact their ability to enjoy special occasions with the same freedom as they did before, as they may not be able to afford to purchase gifts, or even attend some things.

Having someone with dementia sitting at the Christmas or birthday table, or missing out on Christmas because they are living in a residential care facility, can be more difficult for families than a deceased loved one not being there at all.

It is also very difficult to get through the first year of celebrations without someone once they have died, and the loneliness and grief is often heightened at these times, especially the first year after their death. Bob De Marco[27] wrote about his first Christmas without his mother Dotty who died in May 2012 from dementia of the Alzheimer's type, 'I am a little sad and a little lonely. But, the sadness is more than trumped by all the happy memories.'

Festivities can also be stressful and traumatic for the person with dementia. Things like fatigue, noise, loss of the familiar routine, guests they may not remember, not having been able to purchase presents, or not remembering to, and so on, can all cause anxiety and stress.

These times have the potential to intensify the emotional negatives of dementia during and leading up to special occasions, for everyone, and may also increase some of the symptoms in the short term.

Spending time with lots of family or 'old friends' might be more challenging, as there is usually a phrase at the beginning of many of the conversations — sentences too often begin with 'Remember when...' and on the occasions when people with dementia can remember an event or conversation, it isenjoyable. But at the time the person cannot remember, it

---

27   *www.alzheimersreadingroom.com*

may exacerbate the loneliness, the feelings of shame and stigma, and increase the grief and sadness, as well as increase the fear of what's ahead and the feelings of isolation.

It may be easier for the person with dementia to pretend to remember, but not always as easy to participate in extended conversations about events and people, as pretending only works at the very beginning. This is when the feelings of shame, humiliation and embarrassment arise, and, even if they say nothing about it, it may result in their mood or behaviour changing.

Especially at Christmas time, people with dementia who were employed when diagnosed and are no longer working, may be feeling a sense of sadness and loss at no longer being invited to the workplace Christmas parties and other events with colleagues. The experience of dementia often brings with it a loss of some family and friends, and this is more noticeable during times of celebrations and festivities.

Here are some tips that may increase everyone's joy and reduce stress:

» Communicate with family and friends about what works best for everyone.

» Have realistic expectations of what you have the time and energy to do if you are a care partner, and what the person with dementia has the energy, desire and ability to do.

» Ask for help. Often family and friends have no idea what help to offer, and it is always useful for them to be told specifically how they can best assist. Sometimes it is only when you have asked, that others feel comfortable helping.

» Remember, as a care partner, tiredness, frustration and agitation is contagious and will negatively affect the person with dementia. Participating in large social gatherings will also be tiring for people with dementia as they are having to work so much harder to function, cope with noise, and so on.

» Plan somewhere quiet where, if you are the person with dementia, you can disappear for some 'time out' from the celebration; if you are supporting someone with dementia, you may suggest it to them as well.

» As the care partner, it may help you to ask family and

friends to give you some time out so that you can enjoy this time as well.

» Communicate with each other about these things as best you can, before a celebration and throughout.

Here are some pointers to share with friends and family to consider during celebrations:

- asking people with dementia if they remember you can immediately cause feelings of anxiety and a sense of shame if they cannot
- introduce yourself by name, even if you think the person with dementia knows you well; they may have forgotten your name
- showing your hurt or disappointment if they don't recognise you or remember your name might make things worse
- it is more productive not to argue, or tell them they are wrong
- don't actively remind them if someone they don't remember has died, or of someone they don't remember at all
- it may be better if you don't ask them if they remember specific people, things or events but rather talk about people, things or events and let them join in if they can, or wish to
- try not to denigrate, pity or patronise
- remember, they are people, just like you
- don't talk over the person with dementia, or for the person with dementia — give them the time and respect to speak for themselves, no matter how difficult that may be
- don't correct the person with dementia, or talk about them to others in front of them, or undermine them in any way, unless you want to make life more difficult for them, and ultimately for yourself
- accept general comments, and don't ask for detailed explanations
- be prepared for repetition of either a question, or a conversation

- do something practical with the person instead of just talking to them
- always include them in activities
- don't talk about them as if they aren't there
- focus on what they can still do, not the things they cannot do
- focus on the things they want to do, not what you think is best for them
- if you send Christmas or birthday cards to people with dementia, make sure the envelope has your Christian and surname on it, as well as perhaps a family photo or photo of yourself included in the card.

One lady with dementia said:

> *A few years ago, I realised my ability to recall who my friends were was getting bad because when I opened up the Christmas cards, I could not remember who most of them were. The people who included a family photo, or had an address label on the back with both names meant I more easily could work out who they were. For example, getting a card that only says 'Love from Judy', when I know about five Judy's, was no help at all!*

Do your best to have fun, and cope during celebrations, and if you need to disappear to the garden or your room then just do so.

Incontinence

Living with incontinence is difficult at the best of times, but if you have dementia, or are supporting someone with dementia, it can be a bit trickier. There are lots of emotions attached to managing one's own intimate care, and losing the ability to do this will cause stress for everyone.

The progression of dementia almost always means incontinence is inevitable, and although this usually happens later in the disease some reported it happened earlier. Even if you have been a nurse, it presses so many emotional buttons — privacy, disgust, embarrassment, shame, distaste, regret, and so on. It is one thing to wipe the bottom of your child or clean up their soiled underwear, but quite another to do so for a partner or parent. It is also emotionally difficult for older parents to assist with this for an adult child who has dementia, simply because they are adults and it is not natural. If you are the partner of someone with dementia who is becoming incontinent, and are in a sexual or intimate relationship, some will turn away from intimacy and sex, as they fear the embarrassment of incontinence during sex. It is a difficult topic to think about, let alone discuss.

One son said:

> God I hated helping my own mother to wipe her arse, or to clean up her messes before she went into a nursing home. I didn't hate her, but sometimes, it felt like she was doing it on purpose. It is really hard to remember it is the bloody dementia! The only thing that kept me going was knowing she did it for all of us, and well…I really, really love her, even though I miss her the way she used to be…

It is not usually the case that the person with dementia is fully independent in using the toilet on one day, and then the next thing you know is fully incontinent. Incontinence can happen gradually so you will probably have time to adjust, plan and educate yourself about how to manage things. Many do try and hide incontinence though, as people feel ashamed and embarrassed, and many with dementia will try and remove the continence pads.

Once daughter of an older lady with dementia said:

> For me it was a dawning realisation that the messages going to Mum's brain were clearly getting confused. Initially it was a wet bed in the morning every so often, or one day would be fine and then the next she would pull down her pants in the hall and wee, or pull down her pants and sit on the sofa to wee. Initially I got annoyed by this behaviour and I'm not proud of the fact that I did. But I think a lot of it was an underlying denial about what was happening, coupled with an extreme wish for things to be how they

always were — a frequent visitor on the dementia path and one which often causes the most anguish. Of course my mother wasn't consciously setting out to soil the furnishings, in her mind she was simply going to the loo and immediately after she had no memory of having done so. You soon learn the futility of asking why on this very steep learning curve.

Here are some tips to help if the person you support is becoming incontinent:

- » Make sure you always know where the toilets are when you are out — there is now an online national toilet map https://toiletmap.gov.au that you may find useful.
- » Make sure that the person knows how to find the toilet at home — is the problem because he or she is not able to find it or get to it in time, or no longer realises it is a toilet?
- » Make sure that the person recognises where to sit in the toilet, and can find the toilet paper and knows what to do with it.
- » Use a timed toileting regime. You may keep a toileting chart to figure out when the person usually needs to go to the toilet (e.g. when they first wake up, 20 minutes after a cup of tea or a meal) or use a regular toileting schedule, i.e. remind the person to go to the toilet every 2 hours.
- » Give the person with dementia enough time to completely empty their bladder. Sometimes they lose the ability to feel whether they have finished urinating or not and will get up before they have finished, or need to go to the toilet again soon after. A song or a story on the toilet may help with this.
- » Use incontinence pads and change them regularly; this is especially difficult to initiate, as many will find this deeply embarrassing and insulting.
- » Consider installing a bidet to help with washing and drying. If explained properly by the person helping them in the toilet 'you're now going to feel some warm water

washing your bottom', people with dementia are accepting of bidets. The use of bidets may even help people with dementia.

People who work in aged care see residents pulling their pads off, refusing to wear them, ignoring toilets and using the floor. In hospitals and aged care, research tells us that a nurse's minute, 'I'll be back in a minute Mr G.' can take up to an hour. Therefore, if someone does ask you to take them to the toilet and you say I'll be back in a minute, by the time you get back there, it will probably be too late. In residential care, incontinence may be because the person with dementia is not supported to be continent because staff are busy, time poor and task focused. Therefore, the person with dementia may have to wear pads or pull-ups, which is underwear designed to hold continence pads, but which are easier to manage as they pull up like a pair of undies, hence the name.

One older ex-nurse said; 'When I worked in aged care, I remember them sitting on toilets, telling me to go to the toilet myself whilst "refusing" to go themselves. It is difficult to know when someone else needs to go.'

Visiting an incontinence nurse can be very helpful, and they have many suggestions and techniques to help you manage, or to prepare for both urinary and faecal incontinence. Visit the Continence Foundation of Australia for more information here: http://www.continence.org.au. There is also a Continence Aids Payment Scheme where you can apply for financial assistance with continence aids. The application form can be downloaded here: http://www.bladderbowel.gov.au/

Dementia and sexuality

We are all human and the need to be loved and to express love and intimacy, and things such as the desire to dress well and look good do not usually go away with age, or dementia. We all want to look and feel our best, and most adults will still have feelings of intimacy and sexual desire. That is simply a part of being a human being.

The way sexuality is expressed not only differs between heterosexuals and members of the LGBTI communities, it differs with every individual, and also the relationship you are in. How you display intimacy with a friend will be different to how you do that with a sexual partner. Living in an aged care facility, or just being older or having dementia will not automatically mean you will no longer have sexual desires and for some, living in a residential facility may even increase their sexual desires due to the loneliness.

Much has been written about people with dementia in relation to their sexuality, but so far, there is very little written by the cohort it relates to, that is, people with dementia and their sexual partners. Perhaps it is time people with dementia speak up on this topic, as it is personal, intimate, and deeply affects them and their partners. It is not only about inappropriate sexual behaviours in a nursing home or in public, and it is right that people with dementia start to have a voice on this topic.

Just because a person has dementia does not mean they won't want to have sex, although many people with dementia do lose their sexual urges and stop wanting to have sex, due in part to things such as losing their sense of self or the changed relationships brought on by the symptoms of dementia.

Some care partners may even be hoping the type of dementia the person they are supporting has is the type of dementia where they want sex more often, and are perhaps was less inhibited…who knows! Having a conversation about such a personal topic therefore needs to be sensitive and considered.

But sexuality is personal, and an important part of our lives. It is linked to wellbeing, quality of life and to feeling good about ourselves. Most people have a basic human need for it and it is so much more than simply having sex. Something as simple and benign as the way we touch someone's cheek can be sexual, if it is with your partner. Ageing can bring with it physical changes that may mean we have to change the way we express ourselves intimately, but that probably won't change the desire.

People living in facilities (nursing homes) have generally found that wanting sex and intimacy has not been easily accepted, and family members of people with dementia who may have forgotten a spouse and are having a relationship with someone in the home, find this difficult to come to terms with. In an interview on BBC Radio 5 Live's Breakfast program, Eve Carder, who was senior nurse manager at Landermeads Nursing Home, in Chilwell, just outside Nottingham in the UK, said in her experience the staff were regularly faced with tricky dilemmas. Eve said:

One situation in particular involved a lady and a gentleman who were both married before [not to each other] and living with a form of dementia…They believed they were living in a different reality where they were in a relationship together as husband and wife… They would walk round the care home hand in hand, sit on the sofas within the lounge area and cuddle up together…Occasionally they'd lie down on a bed together…Care staff and nursing staff management found the situation very difficult to manage because they saw it as wrong…They saw the gentleman's real wife very distressed. She would come in and openly cry and voice that she couldn't handle seeing her husband with another woman…At one point in a conversation, it was likened to him having an affair.

Eventually, Ms Carder said, his wife had agreed to telephone 20 to 30 minutes before her arrival to allow staff to separate the 'couple'. But that had caused a lot of negative feelings because they had been unable to fully comprehend the situation. Ms Carder said it was important families understood people living with dementia could not rely on logic or reason.

They are overwhelmed with feelings and trying to make sense of the world around them…they will seek comfort, attachment and love in a way that feels right at that time. The man didn't recognise his spouse as his wife anymore, but it didn't mean he didn't connect with her.

Professor Julian Hughes, consultant in old age psychiatry at North Tyneside General Hospital, said in the same interview, changes in sexual behaviour were not always so benign, and can be:

…a form of sexual disinhibition. Mostly this is put down to problems with the front of the brain, which controls our personalities, and if it's damaged by dementia then people can start to do things they wouldn't otherwise normally do. That can show itself in terms of aggression, but it can also show itself in terms of sexual behaviour.

Our brain controls our sexual feelings and inhibitions, and we know that dementia can cause changes in the brain, which affect sexual behaviour, and that these changes are not predictable. Medications can also cause some changes in sexual behaviours. Depending on the part of the brain being affected by dementia (and also the medication being taken), the person may experience:

- changes in the ability to communicate, express and understand can greatly impact sexuality
- changes in what personal boundaries are, or ignoring others' boundaries
- an increased or decreased interest in sex in general, including no interest in sex at all
- a change in sexual sensitivity to the other person's needs, e.g. no desire or need for foreplay anymore
- a change in sexual inhibitions — the person may do or say things that seem out of character or 'inappropriate', such as making sexual advances towards a person who they know is married to someone else
- behaviour that once would have been controlled or only done in private, may now need to be immediately gratified
- unable to consider consequences
- insensitive to the feelings of other family members, including your own spouse.

There is generally a lack of training of staff in dementia, and about sexuality and dementia. It is often difficult for adult children to think about their parents' sexuality, but more so for the adult children of people with dementia to accept that their parents may still want to have sex or be intimate in some way. It is a hugely personal and individual topic, and when it comes to sexuality and dementia, the only people who really know what the experience is, are people with dementia and their (sexual) partners, married, de facto, gay or otherwise.

The changes in sexuality can cause the partners of people with dementia to feel deeply hurt, and can be very emotionally damaging and hard to accept and live with. Having a partner who does not remember you is hard enough, but seeing them then engage in sexual relations, or in other intimate ways with someone else is even more difficult to manage. It is not an easy road for anyone and, importantly, you are not alone. We recommend you seek professional support if you are experiencing any of these or other difficulties with a partner with dementia.

We have also encountered the situation where the person with dementia and their care partner are still married and living together, but are no longer sexually intimate. The care partner then develops a relationship with another person. In this situation, it is not uncommon for the care partner to find some family and friends have great difficulty accepting this as, technically, they are still married to someone else. It is important to always consider what is best for you, and your situation and to be open with your family and friends and ask for their continued acceptance and support.

Always remember, sex is a topic that people often find difficult discussing with their partners, discussing it with strangers may be even more difficult. Everyone is a unique individual, with family history, some with history of sexual abuse you may not know about or they may not remember, as well as cultural and spiritual beliefs that may also form part of their sexual beliefs. Respect, privacy and being non-judgemental are paramount.

'We Are Still Gay' is Australia's first evidenced based study documenting the experiences and needs of LGBT Australians living with dementia. The resource outlines the key identified issues from the research and provides suggested strategies to help meet the needs of LGBT people living with dementia. Read more and download the study and book produced by Val's Café at http://valscafe.org.au

Chapter 9

SERVICES

We encourage you to find out about services, even if you don't need them...

You may be reading this and thinking 'I don't need services...', or 'I'll read this when I need services...' We've encountered many people with dementia and their care partners who don't start using services until they have reached a crisis point. The person with dementia may have lost confidence and become socially isolated, and the care partner is stressed to the point of depression and burnout.

Some people think that they are still managing, and that when things get worse then they will use services. If you are just managing, then services may help you have a better life — give you the opportunities or time to do things that you enjoy and increase your quality of life.

There can be a long wait of months, or even a year, for services in some areas. Hence, making enquiries about services and putting your name on a waiting list, or booking respite care may act as insurance for when you really need the help. The experience of many is that if respite is not planned well in advance and booked in, then when you *really* need it, there are no beds available in a location that suits you.

Even when they realise they need help, some people are not comfortable with the idea of using formal services

Some people are uncomfortable with the idea of a stranger being in their home, or looking after them (or the person with dementia they are supporting). If this is the case, you can make sure that there is a process of building up trust and getting to know the staff providing the service before you give them access to your home or, if you are a care partner, give them full responsibility for the person with dementia.

Accepting you might need external support can be difficult, as many have said they feel it is 'the beginning of the end'. In fact, the reality of accepting services sooner rather than later can mean the difference between everyone living with a better quality of life, and the person with dementia being able to stay in their home.

Well-meaning friends, relatives and health-care professionals often offer their comments and advice about whether you should or should not be accessing services. These comments can sometimes add to the guilt we feel and put us under even more pressure. It is your experience, and you have to do what is best for you and your care partner, if you are the person with dementia, or for you and the person with dementia you are supporting. One size definitely does not fit all.

One of the biggest hurdles people face when services are engaged is having a different person turn up each time, so put some effort into negotiating with the service provider that, where possible, you have the same support worker. One lady with dementia said, 'How would you feel if a stranger came every day to take your clothes off and shower and dress you…oh, and wipe your bottom?!'

One daughter said when asked of her experience in accessing home care, 'Mum found it too difficult to cope with different people coming and taking her different places. She needed someone she could connect to and some continuity.'

With consumer directed care in existence, this is likely to happen less, but many still report it is a major battle and causes the person with dementia and the families and care partners significant distress. No-one feels okay about strangers coming to their home every day.

Support services

Dementia Alliance International

Dementia Alliance International (DAI) is the global voice of dementia, working with the philosophy of 'Nothing about us, without us' and encouraging organisations to act on that philosophy. For too long people with dementia have not been fully included in the very things that affect and matter to them. Dementia Alliance International aims to represent the more than 47.5 million people currently diagnosed with dementia globally.

DAI's vision is simple: A world where a person with dementia continues to be fully valued and fully included.

Dementia Alliance International (DAI) is an advocacy and support group, of, by and for people with dementia. It is a non-profit group of people with dementia from all around the world that seeks to represent, support, and educate others living with the disease, and an organisation that will provide a unified voice in the fight for individual autonomy and improved quality of life.

Membership of Dementia Alliance International is free, and is open and exclusive to anyone with a medical diagnosis of any type of dementia and their membership is now in 35 countries. You can inquire about membership in the list of resources below[28], but it is as simple as going to www.joindai.org.

DAI provides weekly online support groups for people with dementia, and, at the time of writing, Mick Carmody from Brisbane, a Dementia Alliance Board Member and their Global Support Group Manager, hosts and facilitates these weekly online support groups. They are held in time zones suitable to people living in a number of different countries, and everyone with dementia who becomes a member of DAI is welcome to join one of these support groups. Member ship is free.

Support groups help people with dementia beat the isolation of dementia; you will get to learn what fun it is being part of a supportive group of friends, all living with a diagnosis of dementia. There is no need

---

28 *Dementia Alliance International www.joindai.org; www.infodai.org*

to leave home, if you have a way to connect to the internet. Your family support person, or even a paid carer, is able to assist you to attend, but participation is only for people with dementia.

At the time of writing support groups are held in the Australia/New Zealand time zones every Tuesday around lunchtime, and one on a Monday every two weeks. If the time the group in Australia currently runs doesn't suit you, and you have a group of up to 12 people with dementia, you may be able to set one up at a time suitable to you. You can contact DAI about this by email at info@infodai.org

They also have an online support group specifically for people with a diagnosis of Primary Progressive Aphasia as part of their dementia, which allows members to be supported by family and friends to participate.

DAI also provides 24-hour online zoom rooms for a number of different groups, including an exclusive zoom room for people with dementia, one for family care partners and people with dementia, the LGBTI community, and very soon will be hosting support groups for care partners as well. Contact them at info@infodai.org for more information or for the specific login details. Zoom (www.zoom.us) is free to download, and easy to use if you have access to a computer with a camera and the Internet. If you can use Skype, you will easily be able to use zoom.

In the two years since DAI was launched, this global organisation has had an impact on many things, including representation on the World Dementia Council of people with dementia, and representation as a keynote speaker on the world stage at the World Health Organization's First Ministerial Conference on Dementia in Geneva. In this keynote speech, three things people with dementia asked for made it to the WHO final Call to Action. The three of topics of significant importance to people with dementia discussed in Geneva were:

1. That people with dementia have a human right to a more ethical pre- and post-diagnostic pathway of care, including rehabilitation;

2. That people with dementia are treated with the same human rights as everyone else, using the current Disability

Discrimination Acts and the United Nations Convention on the Rights of Persons with Disabilities; and

3. That research does not only focus on a cure, but also on the care of the more than 47 million people currently diagnosed globally.

Dementia Alliance International's global advocacy work is important as the mission to provide direct support for people with dementia, is often lacking. As a collective voice, and with the expertise of Professor Mittler from the UK, DAI is working hard to also ensure the rights of people diagnosed with a dementia, as people with disabilities, are recognised under the *United Nations Convention on the Rights of Persons with Disabilities*. During the UK's Dementia Awareness Week in 2016, they released their first official publication, *Human Rights for People Living with Dementia — Rhetoric to Reality*, available to download here: http://www.dementiaallianceinternational.org/human-rights/.

'Never doubt that a small group of thoughtful committed citizens can change the world — indeed it is the only thing that ever does.' (Margaret Meade)

Alzheimer's Australia

Alzheimer's Australia is the peak advocacy body in Australia for people with dementia (not just Alzheimer's disease) and their care partners and families. They represent the more than 342,800 Australians living with dementia and the estimated 1.2 million Australians involved in their care. They advocate for the needs of people living with all types of dementia, and for their families and care partners, and provide support services, education and information. Alzheimer's Australia is a member of Alzheimer's Disease International.

Alzheimer's Australia also represents, at the national level, the interests of its federation of state and territory members on all matters relating to dementia and carer issues.

Alzheimer's Australia provide Australians with a suite of services and support, currently including:

- care partner support groups
- family care partner education
- counselling
- the living with dementia program — a program of group information and discussion sessions for people with dementia and their care partners and families
- library and information service
- national younger onset dementia key-worker program.

Please note that the Alzheimer's Australia chapters in each state and territory operate independently, so services available in some states are run differently, or are not available in others. When you're navigating the Alzheimer's Australia website it is also important to keep in mind that it is actually multiple state websites which operate relatively autonomously, even though they are under the one banner.

Contact Alzheimer's Australia's national dementia helpline on 1800 100 500 to find out about services in your area. There are lots of useful factsheets and other information on their website https://fightdementia. org.au/

Carers Australia

Carers Australia is the national peak body representing Australia's carers, advocating on behalf of Australia's carers to influence policies and services at a national level. It works collaboratively with partners and its member organisations, the network of state and territory Carers' Associations, to deliver a range of essential national carer services.

Their vision is an Australia that values and supports the contribution that carers make both to the people they care for and to the community as a whole. Their purpose is to work to improve the health, wellbeing, resilience and financial security of carers and to ensure that caring is a shared responsibility of family, community and government.

Alzheimer's Disease International

Alzheimer's Disease International (ADI) is the peak body globally for people with dementia and their care partners and is a worldwide federation of more than 80 Alzheimer's associations. ADI and its member organisations have campaigned to help people live well with dementia and has launched major advocacy and awareness campaigns such as World Alzheimer's Month.

Since 2009, ADI has also published annual *World Alzheimer Reports*, a comprehensive global review on dementia. ADI works locally, by empowering national Alzheimer associations to promote and offer care and support for people with dementia and their carers, whilst working globally to focus attention on the epidemic and campaign for policy change from governments and the World Health Organization.

The ADI website has have a section on their website called I CAN I WILL[29], which is a library of ideas to help people around the world stand up and speak out about Alzheimer's disease and related disorders. People with dementia, their families and others, including professionals, can contribute their stories and shared knowledge.

Aged care services

How to find out about services in your area

Aged care services are funded by the Commonwealth government, but are provided by state governments, local councils, not-for-profit and for-profit organisations. These organisations tender to provide services.

www.myagedcare.gov.au or, within Australia, 1800 200 422 is the Commonwealth government's single point of entry for aged care services. Unfortunately, at the time of writing the website is difficult to navigate, and provides only basic information about the system. What it does contain is a searchable database of services by geographical location. There tend to be more services in cities than in regional and remote areas.

For people in New South Wales see also https://www.hsnet.nsw.gov. au/ which is a searchable website of a variety of services including aged care. The website is run by the Department of Family and Community Services in NSW.

---

29 *http://icaniwill.alz.co.uk/icaniwill.html*

Since the information on my aged care is still improving, the best way currently to find out about services is to phone them directly. Here are some questions to ask:

- what do you do?
- are there any eligibility criteria?
- how long is the waiting list?
- how much will it cost me?
- what is your case manager to client ratio?
- how often will case managers speak to me?
- how often will case managers visit me and review how I am going?

Community and home care services — services while you continue to live in your own home

Services for people with dementia are fragmented, the system is confusing and aged care is undergoing reforms, which means that things are constantly changing. So there is no easy way of finding out what is available in your local area, or how to access these services. Be mindful that there are lengthy waits for some services in some areas.

For historical reasons, Australian community and home care services are grouped into the Commonwealth Home Support Programme (this used to be called HACC or Home and Community Care, except for Victoria and Western Australia where the HACC program continues), Home Care Packages and other programs not directly supported by the Commonwealth.

In theory the home support programme offers lower levels of services for people with lower needs, and home care packages offer co-ordinated higher levels of services for people with greater needs. In reality there is overlap between the amount of services you can get under each type of program.

Commonwealth Home Support Programme

Services provided by the Commonwealth Home Support Programme include:

» Meals-on-wheels: cooked meals delivered to your home.

Some providers offer a wide range of meals including food from different countries. Meals may be delivered warm or chilled depending on your wishes and the provider.

» Domestic assistance: light housework such as vacuuming, mopping, sweeping, dusting, laundry, making beds, ironing, lawn mowing, pet care, spring cleaning.

» Meal assistance: helping you shop, prepare and store food.

» Personal care: helping you have a shower or bath, washing your hair, getting you dressed, going to the toilet, foot and nail care.

» Basic home maintenance: e.g. changing light bulbs or replacing tap washers.

» Equipment to help you stay at home: walkers, wheelchairs, home safety alarms, non-slip bath mats, raised toilet seats, oxygen, nebulisers.

» Basic home safety modifications: e.g. ramps, rails for steps or in the bathroom, alarms.

» Nursing care: a qualified nurse comes to your home to help you manage your health conditions e.g. changing dressings on wounds, monitoring blood pressure or blood sugar, helping manage your medications, helping with continence, skin care, catheter care.

» Allied health support: physiotherapy (exercise to improve mobility, strength and balance), podiatry (foot care), speech pathology (to help with speech, communication, swallowing and eating), occupational therapy (to help you stay independent in doing things for yourself), dietitian (advice on healthy eating).

» Community transport: transport for shopping or to appointments.

» Community visitors: volunteers who visit and offer you social support.

» Care or support during the day: see description of daytime care programs under respite.

» Respite.

In order to obtain a Commonwealth Home Support Programme service, you need to contact the My Aged Care contact centre (1800 200 422) or online at http://www.myagedcare.gov.au/service-finder. Centre staff will ask you a series of questions over the phone, and they may organise a home support assessment by a regional assessment service who will determine your eligibility and make a referral for services.

How much do Commonwealth Home Support Programmes cost?

The Commonwealth Home Support Programme is funded by the Australian government. Some services are free, however there is often a co-payment paid by the service recipient This will differ from service to service and the calculation may be based on your income and assets, as well as the policies of the service organisation. Find out what you may have to pay before signing up to any service.

Home care packages

Home care packages offer case managed services using a consumer directed model. Case management involves having an experienced person assess your needs, help you identify service goals, helps develop a care plan, puts the care plan into place by arranging and coordinating the different services you need, and reviews what is happening regularly. Consumer directed care means that you get to choose what services you want to help you live at home independently and well. Consumer directed care is a shift away from more traditional case management where case managers made decisions about what was best for their clients.

As of 1 January 2016 there were four levels of Home Care Packages, to support people with with basic care needs through to high care needs.

There is also a Dementia Supplement for people with dementia, and a Veterans' supplement for veterans with an accepted mental health condition.

When you are given a home care package, you're allocated a total budget, which is managed for you by the aged care provider. The amount that you contribute to the budget will vary depending on your income but does not differ based on the level of home care package you're getting. The minimum contribution is about $10 a day, plus an income tested fee of up to about $30 a day. For level 1 and 2 packages, if you have a high income your contribution is greater or very similar to the total budget. If this is the case, you may choose to employ your home care services privately.

Managing your home care package

You are free to choose how to spend your home care package budget to help keep you living at home as long as possible — you can't pay for food, rent, utilities or holidays but could use the money to improve the safety of your home, do an exercise program to improve your mobility, or buy a new microwave to heat your food. You can choose what services you want, who delivers the services (e.g. you may want a lady not a man, or you may want someone who speaks a language other than English), what time you get the service, and you can even keep a little of the funds each week in reserve in case of emergencies (in a contingency fund). There is a wide variation between providers in how much actual choice you get within your budget — some providers are more flexible and resourceful in meeting your wishes than others.

You can choose to manage your home care package yourself. This means that you (or your representative) will research and hire services, manage appointments, and you will manage your own budgeting. Most people choose not to have this level of control and responsibility and pay the service provider to undertake these tasks.

When choosing how to spend your home care package, don't feel constrained by the list of services that your home care provider offers. Think about what is really important to you in terms of both your mental and physical wellbeing. For example, we know consumers who have elected to go to aquatherapy once a fortnight, and have their home cleaned every second week instead of weekly. Another consumer 'banked' part of his budget so that he could have a paid care worker help him travel to attend a family wedding.

You should receive a monthly account showing how your government subsidised budget is being spent. Some people have complained that their fee statement is confusing. Consumers have complained that some providers charge high administration and case management fees. These have reportedly been as high as 40% of the total package.

At the time of writing, home care packages are allocated to home care services based on a tender they make to run the packages. This means that if you are not happy with your home care package provider and want to move, you can only do so if another provider in your area has a vacant package. From February 2017, home care packages will be allocated to consumers rather than providers, this means that you will be able to choose which provider you want to provide your home care package.

Home care packages are confusing — http://www.homecaretoday.org.au/consumer is a website that will help you understand how consumer directed home care packages work. This site includes a list of frequently asked questions and is updated to reflect current rules and policies for home care.

Consumer directed care is a new approach. Some case managers have found it difficult shifting to consumer directed care from a more prescriptive case management model (i.e. where the case managers tell you, the client, what they are going to provide you, what time the services they can provide will come, and who they will send to provide the service). If you're aware of these issues it may help you negotiate what you want from your care package. Some case managers:

» Find it hard to balance their perceived duty of care (what they think their client needs) with their client's wishes (what their client say they want). If you find your case manager risk-adverse, ask to be allowed to take calculated risks, and point out the risks to independence or autonomy.

» Find it difficult to talk about financial aspects of the service. Until recently services were fully subsidised by the government and case managers did not have to discuss finances with clients. You need to ask questions and make sure that your case manager fully explains the financial aspects to you.

» Have a conflict between selling services from within their organisation (e.g. home cleaning) and services from outside their organisation (e.g. buying equipment). Make sure that decisions are made in your best interest, rather than to the benefit of the organisation providing your service.

A good case manager should help you put together a care plan to meet your personal goals. The case manager should bring his or her knowledge and experience about paid and free community services (e.g. a visiting service, or a library delivery service) to help you make informed choices about the services that you want and need. A good case manager makes sure that you feel listened to and helps you identify your priorities and goals. He or she gives you education about the options, services and other technologies available that may help in meeting your goals, acts as your advocate, provides emotional support, and leads the team of home care workers and health professionals he or she may arrange to provide services for you. A good case manager is someone who is a good listener and who you can trust to act in your best interest. A good case manager checks in regularly with you to make sure that services are working well, and helps you set new personal goals.

How to access home care packages

You need to be assessed and approved by an Aged Care Assessment Team (ACAT) in order to get a home care package. There can be a wait of months for an ACAT assessment, though if you're in hospital you can get an assessment more quickly. Find out from your ACAT assessor what the process in your area is for getting a home care package once you've got your approval. Some regions keep a centralised waitlist of packages so eventually your number will come up, but most do not have this. This means that the ACAT may refer you to a provider with a long waitlist. Once you have an ACAT approval, you may want to ring local providers, find out about their services and make sure that you are on their waiting, list if there is one.

One daughter said, 'No problems with ACAT, but I am a health care professional, so knew the system.' Many others reported having very a different experience, and one husband said it 'was a nightmare finding out about getting an ACAT for his wife, then being on the never ending waiting list. It wasn't until a crisis that we managed to get one and by then the value of the respite was almost not worth the wait!'

Respite for care partners

Daytime respite

Respite services have been designed to give care partners a break so that they can continue to care for the person with dementia at home for longer. During respite, care partners can focus on their own health and personal needs. However, it is also important that any respite provided, also supports the person with dementia, or both will not get the full benefits. As one wife said:

> *I can't be bothered using this service, as I know my husband hates it, and is bored. The carer follows him around like some sort of puppy, just because the case notes say he might 'wander'! When I return, he is always unhappy and angry, so what's the point?*

Respite can be for a few hours or a few weeks, it can happen in your home, at a centre or in a residential aged care facility (i.e. a nursing home).

Respite at home will involve a care worker coming to your home to look after the person with dementia, or take him or her out for a few hours. Sometimes overnight respite can be arranged.

Respite at a centre where the respite is only during the daytime usually runs from 10am to 3pm. Usually the person with dementia attends weekly (or sometimes more than once a week). Bus transport may be provided and there will be structured group activities and meals at the centre.

People with dementia and their care partners have told us they want less formal alternatives to daytime respite at the earlier stages of dementia. They want to participate in social groups that do activities that are of interest to them. One man with younger onset dementia said, 'If you send me to somewhere called day care, which to me is the place where I used to take my preschool kids, I will become more than one challenging behaviour!'

For example, there is a very successful volunteering programme in WA, where people with dementia are supported through their home care packages to volunteer in the community, in things they like doing. Lifecare and Bunnings ran a project in SA called the Side by Side project, another very successful volunteering program, where the staff at Bunnings received some basic education in dementia and were buddied with a person with dementia who volunteered there. In this project, very soon people with dementia were able to work alone and many said, 'I could have stayed at work if I had been supported like this'.

As our communities become more dementia aware, and the disAbility rights of people with dementia are recognised, then less formal respite could simply mean becoming a member of a fishing or knitting club, or joining a dance group or men's shed. This means the person with dementia would be enjoying their 'respite', and their care partner would not be worrying about whether they were having a good time. Many of the activities like this could be enjoyed by couples or families and friends as well, for example, a Friday night family bowling group where there are plenty of family or friends around to share in supporting the person with dementia. It could also mean a significant reduction in the need for more formal services.

How you talk about daytime respite could be the one difference between the person with dementia being happy to go there, or not. If you present it as a fun activity with a nice group of people that the person will enjoy, the person with dementia will be more likely to attend than if you refer to it as care, day care or respite.

Residential respite

This involves a short temporary stay in a residential aged care facility. Different aged care facilities have different policies about how long the stay can be (i.e. a few nights or up to two weeks).

Care partners often use residential respite when they want to go away on holidays or so that they can get and recover from medical treatments, or to have a regular break in place. It can be helpful if you are feeling like you are becoming burnt out to know that in so many weeks you have some respite planned, and therefore some time out.

Currently, care partners can access 63 days of residential respite each financial year, and you can ask for an assessment if you think that you need extra time.

Some care partners use residential respite to 'try out' an aged care facility to see if it may be suitable for permanent placement.

Emergency respite

This service provides emergency respite 24 hours a day, seven days a week if the care partner needs emergency help looking after the person with dementia, such as because of illness. Emergency respite care can be arranged through the Commonwealth Respite and Carelink Centre on 1800 052 222 during business hours, or 1800 059 059 outside of business hours.

Care partner's guilt

You may feel much less guilty if the person with dementia seems to enjoy their time in respite. If the person with dementia hates going, or appears to be disturbed from the experience on returning home, then some care partners don't find the break that respite gives them worth it.

In July 2012, I retired to care for G 24/7. I soon realised I needed a regular break, so I sought out a day care facility. G, by this time, was at the stage where his behaviour was sometimes difficult; but he was also still in that in-between zone where he was acutely aware of what he was losing. The qualified staff at the centre tried to include him in activities; however, throwing balls in a bucket, drawing with crayons and other simple activities didn't engage G at all; he was annoyed and agitated when I collected him. The crunch came when I had left him at the centre on the fourth visit, and I headed off to the hairdresser; I was almost there after a 30-minute drive when I got the call to say I needed to come and pick up G because they couldn't settle him and he was unsettling the other attendees. I felt betrayed by professionals who I believed knew how to care for my husband and I cried all the way back to the day care centre.

If you struggle with this, remember that care partner burnout and stress is a strong predictor of permanent placement in a residential aged care facility, and also weigh up the longer term benefits to the person with dementia of being able to stay at home because you, the care partner, can have a short break.

Residential aged care

Residential aged care is the government term for permanent group residential care for older people in Australia — most people call these nursing homes. Residential aged care is different from retirement villages where people live in their own units or apartments. Retirement villages are not government funded (though you may find retirement village units and nursing homes located in the one development).

Going into residential aged care

So how do you pack a lifetime into a small suitcase? This is something many must face, and Kate Swaffer was been personally confronted with this a few times. When packing up for her father-in-law to leave his home to live in a small room in a residential care facility, packing his life into one or two suitcases to enter aged care was confronting and sad, and he hated it, 'Every single day he said he felt locked in prison. Every single day we felt as if we had been his jailer'.

Another time, as a legal guardian for Michael, a close family friend, Kate packed for his move into residential care. After Michael's death, packing a suitcase of his personal and special belongings to take to his family in the UK, it was incredibly difficult to select items from his 57 years to pack into one small suitcase. As she lifted the small suitcase at the airport for weighing and loading for the trip, the fragility of life struck her, and the visual of an actual suitcase, full of a very big life was overwhelmingly sad.

Kate Swaffer's mother-in-law died in her own home, and this is perhaps the greatest gift you can give anyone when they are dying. No need to pack a big life into a small suitcase, and not once did she have to endure the feeling she had been locked in jail. This is not always possible, although, as mentioned earlier, seeking support as a care partner earlier rather than waiting for a crisis may be one of the things that enables someone with dementia to be cared for at home until death.

We talked to many care partners, and heard over and over negative stories of residential aged care. We heard about untrained, neglectful staff, or not enough staff, very few appropriate activities, terrible food, poor clinical care and high rates of chemical restraint (i.e. antipsychotic medication). One has to wonder why this is. We also heard of some good and positive experiences in residential aged care, and have hope that these are becoming the norm, as the aged care sector is undergoing significant reform.

One care partner told us:

> *For the past 15 years I've tried my best to learn and understand from my Mom's experience of living with dementia. She is now 92, and for the last four years has resided in a memory assisted living facility. Like many of these institutions it does an adequate job...but that's it. I've toured many of them and adequate is the best you can say. Real care, understanding and respect for those living with dementia is not the standard model of care here or anywhere that I know of...except perhaps a few facilities for the fabulously well-to-do.*

Many in the aged care sector are working hard to improve things in aged and dementia care, and there is hope that in the future, most facilities will be places we all would be happy to live in. This sector is faced with many challenges: stigma against the industry, complicated funding systems, high levels of paperwork and compliance, lower paid work force, and ongoing State and Federal government changes.

One of the greatest challenges is the low rates of pay. Aged care nurses are paid lower wages than nurses in comparable positions in hospitals, and in many states, staff at the zoo are paid more to clean out the animal cages than we pay our aged care staff. We need an aged care and dementia care industry that is paid well, and appreciates the incredible people who work in it.

Nobody usually chooses to go into aged care or chooses to put someone they love into aged care. The decision is made because circumstances mean that the person with dementia can no longer be cared for at home, either because he or she is unsafe, the amount of care needed is too great, or because continuing to care for the person at home will damage the care partner's health.

We also heard stories of older people, without dementia, choosing to move into low care residential facilities, as the effort of living at home was too much for them, and they didn't feel like going through the process of engaging with service providers at home. Their families had advised against it, but they didn't wish to take the risk of 'being a burden to their families' if they became unwell.

One lady said, 'I wish I'd done it years ago. It's better than sliced bread. Someone cooks and cleans for me, and even does the washing!'

This lady was still driving and even had her own car there, so was able to continue living a reasonably independent lifestyle, but with a lot of support. In doing this she also significantly reduced her loneliness, as she had been living alone, with very few of her lifelong friends still alive, but the many of the stories we heard were less positive than that.

One aged care provider said, 'All too often we assume that the person is either independent to keep doing it themselves, or no longer capable or interested, so we reduce their world for safety or by neglect.'

Dignity in Care Australia

The Dignity in Care program was developed in the UK and launched there in 2006 and aims to put dignity and respect at the heart of UK care services. Dignity in Care Australia was brought to Adelaide by a senior consultant geriatrician, Dr Faizel Ibrahim. Dignity in Care Australia was launched in early 2011 at The Queen Elizabeth Hospital (TQEH), with Maggie Beer as the patron; the program started with 300 enthusiastic champions, and now has over 1000. It is now being rolled out to the whole of South Australian Health, some residential care facilities in South Australia, as well as a large number of hospitals throughout Australia. The Dignity in Care program aims to change the culture of health services by reinforcing the importance of treating patients with dignity and respect.

When people with dementia are always treated with dignity and respect by implementing the 10 Dignity in Care Principles, it leads to a huge change in the way the person experiences living with dementia. It can also positively transform the lives of their care partners and families.

The core principles work positively towards reducing behaviour and mood changes in dementia, and we suggest you evaluate any residential facility you might be considering against them. They relate not only to the actual practical care provided but the quality of the food and the cultural and spiritual needs of the person. If care is to be person centred, then these principles must also be in place.

The ten Dignity in Care Principles:

1. Zero tolerance of all forms of abuse.

2. Support people with the same respect you would want for yourself or a member of your family.

3. Treat each person as an individual by offering a personalised service.

4. Enable people to maintain the maximum possible level of independence, choice and control.

5. Listen and support people to express their needs and wants.

6. Respect people's right to privacy.

7. Ensure people feel able to complain without fear of retribution.

8. Engage with family members and carers as care partners.

9. Assist people to maintain confidence and positive self-esteem.

10. Act to alleviate people's loneliness and isolation.

Choosing a residential aged care facility

There is no 'right time' to start looking at residential aged care facilities. Some people with dementia start looking early because they want to be involved in the decision about where they will stay in the future, and some carers look early 'just in case', as popular facilities can have long waiting lists. Others don't look until the person can no longer be looked after at home.

Be aware that choosing a residential aged care facility can take some time. It takes time to visit each facility and to weigh and compare options, including costs, distance from carers, and staffing and care quality.

Make a list of criteria that you want from the residential care facility before you start looking. Travel time from your family, a single room and a home-like environment may be important to you. Language spoken and culture may also be important. Families are sometimes seduced by fancy architecture or beautiful furnishings and don't take time to think about whether the environment is best for the person with dementia. Some people may not feel that a five-star hotel luxury setting feels like 'home'.

It is really important to physically visit aged care facilities that you are considering. The person showing you around will be doing their sales pitch, so make sure you ask plenty of questions.

Ask about the care and activities that are provided — don't just take the word of the glossy brochures. You may sometimes be shown an activity calendar — ask if the activities all run as programs (in some places what happens and the calendar don't match). Talk to the staff about which activities would suit people with mild, moderate or severe stages of dementia. Usually, not all activities are suitable for everyone, so make sure there are activities that the person who may live there may enjoy. For example, if the person enjoys walking, then a gentle, chair-based stretching exercise program may not meet the person's need to move and give them enough aerobic exercise and they may like being part of a walking group of fitter residents.

It is also important to take time to watch what the residents are doing within the facility — are they happy and busy, or just staring into space with the television blaring. If you were there all day, seven days a week do you think you could be happy and occupied? If you can observe a meal, what is the food like? What is the atmosphere during the meal like? As you watch the staff interact with residents within the facility, consider whether the dignity in care principles (see above) are being met.

Another issue is to think about how the person who is going to live there will 'fit' within the group he or she will be living with. Units within a nursing home are often very different. Residents are usually grouped according to level of care needs (low or high), but may also be grouped according to their level of dementia. Try and imagine what it would be like for the person who is going to live there to live with the other residents. Someone with dementia may find themselves in a secure dementia unit with lots of other people with dementia who behave in ways which are confusing or distressing. Or they may find themself with other people with dementia who have reasonable social skills and enjoy doing the same things that they do, so they may make friends. Fitting in seems to be most difficult for people with dementia who are placed with others who have much poorer cognitive and social skills, so try to avoid this.

The knowledge and skills of the staff in interpreting, understanding and responding to the behaviour and mood of the person with dementia are critical.

Other important factors to consider when choosing a residential care facility are if it will meet the language, cultural and spiritual needs of the person entering the facility, including if the food is culturally appropriate, and also spiritually appropriate at times, such as, a Muslim during Ramadan or a practising Catholic at Easter. Even dress codes of the staff and other residents may seem offensive to people from some cultures and they may not be comfortable being amongst mixed sexes at certain times. Aboriginal Australians have different cultural needs as well as lifestyle, and may not wish to live in an institutional style, let alone sleep in a bed or inside at all. We live in a very multicultural Australia, and the sector promises person centred care, therefore, you have every right to look for it and demand it.

One care partner described how facility staff understood and reacted to behaviour, which could have been construed as undesirable:

One puzzling thing for the staff was that he (the person with dementia) would often take the visitors' sign-in book, take one of the flat cushions off a chair, unzip the cover and put the sign-in book in the cushion, carrying it around with him under his arm. Sometimes he would take the book and — you guessed it — scribble notes on the pages. When the lovely diversional therapist and I had a chat, she had a brilliant idea. She provided a large journal and some pens and I brought in a briefcase for her. So, she started having sit-down meetings with him during which he wrote lots of notes! How brilliant was that! This for me is just one of the finest examples of finding an activity that is totally suited to the person.

Talk to facility staff about the behaviours and mood of the person with dementia, and ask how they will handle them. Try and talk to on-the-floor staff, as the floor staff actually involved in care may not share the attitudes or meet the standards being promised by the senior staff doing the facility tour. Find out what the facility's attitudes towards family care partners are — will the facility keep working with you as a partner in care, or see you as an inconvenience? Some people have been told not to visit for the first few weeks to allow the new resident to 'settle in'; this seems to disregard both the resident's and care partner's feelings.

You may want to ask what the ratio of floor staff to residents is, and the ratio of registered nurses to residents, and if they have registered nurses on during every shift, not just on call. Ask what their attitude to palliative care is, and to adhering to a person's end of life wishes, as many have reported experiences of a mother or father who did not wish to have their life prolonged being sent to hospital without the family's permission, to administer intravenous antibiotics for pneumonia. If the pneumonia was caused by the later stages of the dementia, and the wish was that this type of intervention should not occur, then it has been forced upon the person against their will, and without permission. We have seen and heard of many examples of this happening.

No nurse or paid carer wants someone they care for, and have probably formed a close bond with, to die but at the end of life that is what will happen, and you need to know your end of life wishes will be respected and acted upon.

Here is some advice from a care partner asked about choosing a residential aged care facility:

> *Firstly, it is extremely hard to find a bed. Secondly, I believe it's crucial to try not to be influenced by the glossy brochures, the beautiful artworks on the walls and the modern lounges and guest areas. The primary criterion in selecting permanent residential care is the quality of care practised and the ability of care workers to relate to the resident as a person and not as a disease; to respect them, engage with them on a personal level and enable them to experience the maximum quality of life in care of which they are capable.*

Kate wrote an article, 'What people with dementia want from residential care homes'[30] based on her experience of living with younger onset dementia, as a past care partner and from feedback gathered during interviews and focus groups with people with dementia around Australia and the following is a list of what consumers said they wanted:

- re-ablement
- exercise, lifestyle and diet — all important to quality of life and wellbeing
- supports and strategies for disAbilities to enable independence
- lots of space — inside and outside
- own keys or access to an outside area, even if the front door is locked
- Recreational areas for walking, birds, natural environments
- created environment
- absence of apparent barriers/walls
- screen for audio/visual entertainment (communal get-togethers)

---

30 K Swaffer, 'What People With Dementia Want From Residential Care Homes', Australian Journal of Dementia Care, *vol. 5, no 3, 2016, pp. 21–23*

- open access to the outside world (even if chaperoned)
- outside community coming in
- family can stay overnight in privacy
- personalised furnishings (everybody wants their own style)
- LGBTI friends can stay
- resident autonomy and power — ideas and suggestions are taken seriously and can influence services such as how many settings for dinner and getting people involved in the process
- use of technology
- access to walking groups, dancing classes, normal exercise, gyms, social recreational sport (fishing, bowls, etc. in the community)
- onsite rehabilitation and gymnasium, with sports physiologists or physiotherapists to assist.

She also wrote:

When looking for residential care for ourselves or someone we support, there are four key questions we are often told to ask and that are considered specific to the needs of the person moving into care:

1. Is the facility providing culturally appropriate care and services, including culturally appropriate food?

2. Are the person's relatives and friends encouraged to be involved?

3. What non-medication therapies do they use in their facility? What forms of restraint are used, including chemical and physical? How do they engage residents throughout the day?

4. How do they support residents and families through the end-of-life care process, and do they engage with or bring in specialist community palliative care teams?

One very important point missing in this list of considerations, is if the facility has been built or renovated using the dementia enabling environments principles, as this is becoming a human rights issue for residents in aged and dementia care. Easy access to the outside, not feeling locked in, the ability to engage in everyday lifestyle activities like helping with the washing or cooking, and today, smaller home-style accommodation are...provided for a few in the sector, and will be demanded in the future. Institutional living is being seen as no longer a suitable way to provide the last home a person will ever reside in, at least from the consumer's perspective, which is becoming increasingly central to the provision of any care.

The cost of residential aged care

The Australian government subsidises residential aged care, but funding arrangements are complex. You pay:

» An income and asset tested accommodation payment (you can pay this as a lump sum, or as regular payments, like rent), this may range from $200,000 to over $1 million depending on the location of the home, the size of the room and other considerations such as a water view. If you pay a lump sum up front, the facility will deduct a retention amount each month (this differs depending on the size of the payment), and when the person leaves the facility the remainder will be returned to them (or to their estate if they pass away). Some carer partners have successfully negotiated lower bonds.

» A basic daily services fee (85% of the single pension rate (about $50 a day) which increases twice a year in alignment with pension increases).

» An income and asset tested additional fee.

» You can also choose to pay for extra services — these will differ depending on the facility and include items such as a daily newspaper or cable television, hairdressing and manicures.

There is a residential fee calculator on www.myagedcare.gov.au. You will need information about your assets and income before you can complete it, and it is not easy to complete. Consider seeking financial advice from a residential aged care finance expert before making financial decisions such as whether to sell your home to fund your aged care admission.

Private aged care services

You may consider paying privately for aged care services rather than using government subsidised services, especially if you are someone who will pay a greater contribution towards government services because you have greater income or assets. There are private home care and nursing services as well as residential aged care services (though there are fewer of these).

You may have more control over the services you receive if you pay privately for services. Be aware however that accreditation and quality controls do not apply in the same way to private services, so do your homework before signing up to a service to ensure that they provide good quality care.

Hospitals

Preparing and planning for a hospital stay

People with dementia are more likely to be hospitalised, have longer admissions for the same illness and have higher costs of care than people of a similar age without dementia.

There will probably be occasions when the person with dementia or their care partner has to go to hospital. Emergencies, accidents and many other things can happen that could mean a hospital stay and, if you are prepared in advance, it will be a lot less stressful for everyone. It will also make the job of the hospital staff much easier, and ensure you have the best chance of being optimally cared for.

Keep a hospital bag packed including details such as Medicare numbers, private health care number, medication lists, and health care needs for both the person with dementia and their care partner, as well as contact information for relatives or friends. Other important documents that may be needed are your enduring power of attorney, enduring power of guardianship, as well as Advanced Care Directives (see Chapter 5).

If you are someone with dementia, try to plan what you may do if your care partner needs to go to hospital. If the person with dementia is unable to live alone, their care partner will need to have arrangements made for someone either to support them in the home, or somewhere where they feel most comfortable. Speak to the family member, friends or neighbours and get in principle agreement beforehand, so that it will be easier if an emergency arises. If a care partner is ill and hospitalised, it may affect the person's experience or expression of dementia and their ability to cope. Having arrangements made in anticipation may help minimise stress.

Keep a list at home of important contacts and other information in a clearly named folder, and store it somewhere easily found. Material in the folder could include details for:

- neighbours
- plumber
- electrician
- taxi service
- care services (in case you need to cancel)
- hospital or clinic
- GP
- dentist
- medical specialists
- other medical practitioners you see
- solicitor
- contact at the bank or building society.

It is also advisable to include:

- banking and credit card details — remember you may need passwords
- list of medications
- copy of legal documents such as Power of Attorney or

Advance Care Directives
- a cash float in the overnight bag may also be helpful
- a copy of the completed Alzheimer's UK 'This is me' brochure (see below), or the ACD form being used in South Australia
- a copy of the Alzheimer's Australia 'Talk to Me' brochure on communicating with people with dementia to give to hospital staff
- sheet with dietary needs and allergies, including cultural or spiritual needs.

Keep a list of relevant contacts in your phone as well as in this folder. Label the contacts so it is obvious who they as, if you are in a panic during an emergency this information may not come to mind, e.g. Alan Black Dad's GP, George Dad's plumber, rather than just Alan Black and George.

Essentials to take to hospital are:
- a change of clothes
- underwear
- incontinence or sanitary pads if used (the ward may not have the same brand product you are used to)
- nightwear (the ward will have gowns, but not nightwear)
- dressing gown and slippers
- toiletries, including tissues
- makeup
- a travel-sized hair dryer and brushes or a comb
- reading glasses, hearing aids, spare batteries if needed for hearing aids
- dentures, if used, and denture cleaner
- medication (try to keep in the boxes they came in with instructions), or a list, or the Webster packs if they are in use
- recent copy of any prescriptions from your GP
- mobility aids, e.g. walking stick, walking frame
- a preferred pillow

- some familiar personal items which may make you comfortable, e.g. photos, favourite drinks, sweets, biscuits, favourite perfume or scent
- contact details for family members and next of kin.

Hospitals and people with dementia

Hospitals can be stressful at the best of times, and may cause additional distress to a person with dementia because of the unfamiliar surroundings; the high levels of noise and bustle of a busy ward may disorient them and simple things like finding a bathroom may become more difficult than usual. Hospitals are not dementia enabling and rarely have good signage, so it may help to make some signs if the person with dementia's stay is longer than a couple of days.

Some hospital staff in Australia have had minimal or no training on the care of people with dementia. Make sure that hospital staff are aware that the person has a diagnosis of dementia. Explain how the dementia may impact on the way the person thinks, behaves and communicates. The care partner may have to advocate for the person with dementia and offer suggestions to staff to help them understand and manage behaviours.

The Alzheimer's Society UK have a simple two-page document called 'This is Me'. This gives hospital staff important information about the person with dementia to help see the person as an individual and provide person-centred care. We suggest you print and complete this in advance at www.alzheimers.org.uk/thisisme, and give it to hospital staff to include in medical notes, or put together your own.

The care partner's presence will help keep the person with dementia calmer. Spend time with them — read to them, play music, talk, or just hold their hand. You may be able to help with the person's personal care, such as helping with their meals, or supporting them to go to the toilet. If the person with dementia finds it stressful or disturbing to be in a busy noisy ward, try and find a quiet room (there may even be a courtyard) where you can get away from the noise and people.

Complaints

If you are unhappy with any aspect of your care, or the care of the person you are supporting, talk to the nurse manager or your doctor at the hospital. You may be able to use the dignity in care principles to support your complaint. There is also a formal complaint system in place if this is required. You should not have to accept poor care.

One important point to consider when making complaints is to make them in a way that allows you to maintain good relationships with the staff on site, as that is important for all future success and positive experiences for you all. They are usually doing the very best they can, often under stringent funding restrictions and low patient-to-staff ratios.

Being a care partner of someone in residential aged care

A care partner doesn't stop caring once a person with dementia enters residential care. The aged care facility may take over the physical aspects of care, but family and friends continue to be really important for the person's emotional wellbeing, giving love and support to the person and keeping them company. Your visits (even if the person doesn't seem to remember them afterwards) are really important — the feelings of security and happiness will remain, even if the episode is forgotten.

Family and friends need to be advocates for the person with dementia. Help the aged care staff get to know the person with dementia — the more they see them as a person, the more individualised care they can provide. Bring in old photos, talk about what he or she did in their life, and tell staff what they like doing now. Bring in a DVD of their favourite movie, or a CD of their favourite music. If there are activities that they like doing, make sure that staff know what these are.

Insist on being part of the care planning process, and ask to be involved during care plan reviews. If you observe staff treating the person with dementia in a way that you're not comfortable with, discuss this with management. Try to phrase the complaint positively, rather than blaming the staff member, suggest how you would like the person to be treated. You can cite the dignity in care principles as best practice dementia care, if these help support your point. It can be difficult to complain, as you don't want the person with dementia to be treated even more badly because you've complained. However, unless you speak up things will not improve.

You could also consider attending resident or family meetings, or even joining the resident/family committee. These are other opportunities in which you can voice suggestions for how care can be improved.

Volunteering in some way at the site is also helpful, for example working in the cafe or a 'walking for residents program', as this creates positive interaction.

This is what one family care partner said when asked what advice would she give to other families thinking about on residential care:

> It depends; are you going to dump and run or are you going to put in all the work required to make sure your loved one is treated well? If you choose the latter then expect it to be really hard work, but possibly you will gain a new family and you will be the wiser for it all. Perhaps you get as much as you give. I made it my second home, everyone knew Mum and me and I made sure I had good relationships with the staff and residents as I thought that was in Mum's best interests. While you need to work hard to make sure your loved one has good care, you can't possible criticise and critique everything that happens as you will destroy yourself and possibly those who are trying to do their best. Be appreciative every day, give lots of thanks, give chocolates and gifts at special times of the year, participate in the life of the facility, attend birthday parties etc. join in.

Dental care and dementia

Good dental hygiene plays an important role in the wellbeing of everyone, and therefore also a person with dementia. At the very early stages someone with dementia will be able to manage their own dental hygiene and care and this is the time that you have an opportunity to put some things into place, which will serve you well over the next few years.

Visit the dentist to discuss future appointments and ensure the dental practice understands what dementia is, how dementia could impact on dental health and how dental care needs to be managed in future. Even though in the early stages the person with dementia may be able to maintain their dental hygiene well using a regular toothbrush, this is the time it may be worth introducing an electric toothbrush, as that will make things a little easier later on. Some care partners may find they eventually need to prompt the person with dementia to clean their teeth, others may find it becomes an obsessive behaviour. As always, it is individual.

As dementia progresses, some people with dementia may forget how to clean their teeth; carers may be able to stimulate this memory by standing in front of their relative and brushing their own teeth, whilst the person with dementia copies them. At some stage the care partner may need to take on the task of teeth cleaning. Your dentist or the dental hygienist will be able to show you how to do this properly, being mindful of the spatial awareness of the person with dementia and their anxiety around having someone else do this for them. If you are supporting someone with dementia to clean their teeth, or need to do it for them, this is a good resource that gives some general guidelines and tips: http://unfrazzledcare.com/family-caregiving-just-how-do-you-brush-someone-elses-teeth/

Regular dental checks are important, including in residential aged care. It may be more difficult to get this done in aged care facilities, as many facilities do not have dental services come to them. Some nursing homes neglect dental care, and care partners need to monitor this. Sometimes, hospitals fail in providing adequate dental care for people with dementia as well.

Visits and consultations to the dentist can pose challenges for the person with dementia. If you are the care partner and will be attending with the person with dementia, you will need to let the practice know when you make the appointment.

If you have Power of Attorney, you should also let the practice know this when you call — it will make things easier as there are issues around confidentiality and dignity and the practice will need to be reassured that the person you are accompanying has given their consent. Always check that this is recorded in the person with dementia's notes.

If you don't have Power of Attorney, once you reach the practice and are shown into the consulting room, you should discuss your role with the staff and the person with dementia you are supporting, so that you can demonstrate that the patient is in agreement with you being there and has given their consent. This can be much more difficult without formal Power of Attorney or Power of Guardianship documentation.

If the dental practice has a noisy waiting room, especially if you can hear dental drills and other medical noises, it may be sensible to wait outside in the car. When being treated, some people with dementia may find it difficult to sit still for long periods, or are frightened or upset by the noise or smells of dental equipment, or find it difficult to keep their mouth open for long periods. Be kind and gentle and reassure the person with dementia that you will stay with them, if that is their wish. If it helps, hold the person's hand, you may also be able to play them music using headphones and an iPod or phone.

Chapter 10

ADDITIONAL GROUPS WHO MAY HAVE OTHER NEEDS

Living alone with dementia

Where to live, and who to live with is an important consideration for everyone. In this section we reflect on people who are living alone with dementia.

We estimate that about a third of people living with dementia at home live alone. In the earlier phases of living with a diagnosis of dementia, there can be a positives and negatives of living alone versus living with a partner or others family members or friends. We have talked to people and seen people in different living arrangements, and, to begin this section, we share some lived experiences. As dementia progresses and cognitive capacity and functioning and physical abilities deteriorate, and other issues such as visual, spatial and swallowing difficulties increase, living alone often becomes unsafe. If living with family is not an option, then residential care of some kind is required.

Dr Judy Galvin, a retired academic who is living in Australia, has written a short article for this book on her personal experience of living alone with a dementia for more than ten years.

'For those without a Voice — Living Alone with Alzheimer's', by Dr Judy Galvin

There is a pathway of loss beginning with the words — 'You do have Alzheimer's.' Suddenly your world changes and you walk away wondering who you are now, alone in the realisation that the pathway you now walk will diminish ahead of you, and the substance, the meaning of your life, recede with it. And who is there to tell? You make your way home, alone.

Diagnosis is a passport to a new life, a new identity. You are no longer Dr Judith Galvin — 'I am Judy, and I have Alzheimer's' is the nametag you wear now. Fewer people will want to know you; some old friends forget you. You will soon become redundant. This is now who you are — a person left wondering, fumbling for words, losing identity, with no shared future.

Because you still can, you embrace this new identity and, like a refugee, create a new social network with people like yourself, people with Alzheimer's, their carers and services — the Alzheimer's community. You read their books and follow their websites. You attend the 'Living with Memory Loss' course, information seminars, Cafe Connect outings, and the Memory Loss Centre library.

But none of the people you ever see there are single. Sitting alone among the coupled presence of others, you keep asking yourself — 'Where are my fellow travellers? Where are the others who live alone with dementia?' They are notable by their absence — outsiders, abandoned, without voice, without an advocate — 'missing in action'.

So you lobby on behalf of 'those without a voice'. As a member of Dementia Advisory Committees, you drown in submissions, protesting their absence and consequent neglect, not only from support programs, but from dementia research, national data, planning documents and services. All fail to acknowledge their very existence and their need to be monitored and supported, in a different way.

Time has revealed the life situations of those both with, and without a carer. You have witnessed the depth of dedication, commitment and contribution of carers; and, in equal measure, the frightening dilemma created by their absence; or *presumed existence*, lacking definition, for those who live alone.

Though I live alone and do have Alzheimer's, I am fortunate that, for me, diagnosis came early, medication has been effective, and the disease has progressed slowly. There has been time to plan ahead, develop strategies to function better, select activities I can manage, and to maintain my close relationships. But time is a rare blessing. For the majority, insight and management is more elusive.

Loss often proceeds too quickly, overtaking capabilities till one is left helpless, without voice, without function, stripped of all memory, intellect, and personality. Robbed of autonomy, one struggles to retain, to give expression to a semblance of one's identity, one's past, of the person who remains. For those without a voice and without an advocate — those who live alone, irrespective of the rate of change, the easy solution has been, and remains, institutionalisation, much earlier than necessary.

People who live alone are systematically *excluded* from a national dialogue that begins with research, then data for planning appropriate support. The consequence is breakdown in their pathway of care, resulting in premature institutionalisation, very costly to government, and an abuse of human rights. As an advocate my goal has been *inclusion* through structural change; for an *advocate/monitor* role to enable equity of access to quality support, along the pathway of care, following diagnosis.

How can a person living alone with dementia, without the advocate/monitor (or carer) access 'Consumer Directed Care'? How can they find the *promised land* via the Gateway to Care, along an Internet minefield? Who will take them to where they need to go? Who will protect them from accident and misadventure, note a breakdown in hygiene, nutrition or care? And who will ever know of their physical abuse, or financial abuse, at home, or in a nursing home? Who will ever know?

And Is Anybody Listening?

There is another perspective to consider for people living alone with a dementia, and many of the people interviewed for this book have talked about the benefits of living alone. As always, there are two sides of a coin, and Wendy Mitchell who lives alone in the UK gives us another viewpoint.[31]

Training and support for couples in the practicalities is something else that's sadly lacking post diagnosis. It got me thinking about how lucky I am, in many ways, to live alone. It's a family joke that my eldest daughter, Sarah, moved out of my home on the day I was diagnosed. This wasn't due to Sarah 'running for the hills' at the prospect of what lay ahead, but a happily made decision to set up home with her partner.

However, it was actually a blessing in disguise. When you live with someone, it's quite natural for one to move things around, tidy up, be messy — all of which would be unhelpful for me.

It's human nature to do things for the kindest of reasons but which would annoy the hell out of me in reality.

I'm an independent kinda person who likes to be left to her own devices. I used to be really tidy and not have papers everywhere, however, if I now file papers away, they no longer exist. So on my stairs at the moment are various bits of paperwork where the subject matter is still outstanding. All the paperwork around me moving house is there — because I haven't moved yet; all the paperwork that would normally get filed away because I would remember to deal with it is still there until it's happened — then it can be filed away.

I'm fortunate in so far as I was always an organised person so I haven't had to learn that new skill.

The worktops in my kitchen are far more cluttered than they ever used to be. Each week I lay out paperwork that I need for the coming week. My calendar gets stuffed with paperwork relevant for each month so I don't forget to deal with it. Notes lay strewn everywhere to remind me to do things or as a reminder that something is happening.

---

31 *https://whichmeamitoday.wordpress.com/blog*

If there was someone else living in the house, it may become impractical or be seen as a nuisance, maybe annoying or something may get moved accidentally — all of which would lead to confusion.

- I don't have someone rushing me or questioning why I can't remember something
- I don't have to give excuses or reasons for my action
- I don't have someone doing things for me because it's quicker
- I don't have someone fussing when I'm having a bad day
- I don't have someone urging me to eat when I'm not hungry
- I don't have to think whether I've upset them
- I don't have to worry that I'm having to do things differently
- I don't have to worry about being slow
- I don't have anyone correcting me when I get the wrong word or date or name
- I don't feel like I'm letting anyone down
- I don't have to justify why I'm behaving as I am.

However, there are things that I miss

- I don't have that hug available when things go wrong
- I don't have someone to help jog my memory
- I don't have that support when I find things difficult
- I don't have that back up brain to remind me
- I don't have the constant company
- I don't have that someone to laugh with
- I don't have someone to switch off the cooker when I forget.

Often there seems to be a tug-of-war within households where the person has a partner or other family members living with them, with both parties pulling at the same problem but in opposite directions. Most often this is unhelpful to both parties, and causes friction and unhappiness.

It may be easier for some to live alone in the earlier phases of dementia but, later on, this results in the person almost always forced into residential care.

If you are reading this, and are a friend or family member of a person living alone, remember living alone can be lonely even when someone is well. As the friends drop away after the diagnosis and isolation increases, ,do make a special effort to support your friend or family member who is living alone with dementia.

One man with dementia who lives alone said, 'I have always liked living alone, but one thing I used to hate was eating on my own. Now I have trouble cooking, so that sorted that out!'

If you are lonely, and no longer can drive, and on top of that cannot safely cook, or can't remember how to cook, these are the times friends and family become most important.

Common issues for people with dementia living alone are:
- being able to manage their medication
- risk of malnutrition
- home safety
- feeling lonely or isolated
- being able to contact someone if you fall or have an accident or medical incident and having someone to check up on you regularly in case this occurs
- not being scammed or financially abused.

Moving in with a partner or family

If you're living alone with dementia when diagnosed, you may consider or be pressured into moving in with your care partner. Sometimes, family and friends will tell you if you don't move in with them, they will 'have to make you go into care' and it can be a very difficult time for families with much angst. If this happens, and you agree to move in with someone, here are some considerations that the person with dementia may want to discuss or the care partner may want to ask:
  » The person with dementia may want to remain as independent as possible — what things are essential for you to keep doing yourself? What things would you like to keep doing for yourself?

» The person with dementia may want to contribute to the joint household — how can you do this either financially or in terms of doing things around the house?
» What things do you expect to do together as a household, for example what meals will you eat together, what activities will you do?
» The person with dementia and care partner may wish to have a separate areas for relaxing, for example, somewhere to watch your own TV or listen to your own music, or entertain your own guests.

Younger Onset Dementia (YOD)

Younger Onset Dementia (YOD) (sometimes referred to as early onset dementia) refers to dementia where symptoms started when the person was under the age of 65 years. Younger onset dementia has gradually become the preferred term because early onset of dementia can also refer to people of any age.

In 2016, it is estimated that there are approximately 25,100[32] people with younger onset dementia in Australia. This represents approximately 7% of all those with dementia.

Younger onset dementia may be caused by a number of different types of dementia including Alzheimer's disease, vascular dementia, frontotemporal lobar degeneration, alcohol abuse, Parkinson's disease, Lewy bodies, Huntington's disease and other neurological conditions.

People with YOD have very different needs from older people with dementia. They may have young partners and children still living at home, are often still working and driving, and may have significant financial commitments. The lack of age appropriate services has been a big barrier to accessing care. Younger people have had to access services through the aged care system, which can be very difficult as many are simply told, 'You are too young to access services.'

---

32 *https://fightdementia.org.au/about-dementia/statistics*

The impact of a diagnosis of YOD

Although the symptoms of dementia are similar, whatever a person's age, the impact of these symptoms on younger people with dementia is different to those over the age of 65. The following is a list of impacts on YOD which may be greater than people with late onset dementia.

Greater impact on lifestyle and finances

- » Greater chance of Prescribed Disengagement.
- » Usually still in paid employment.
- » Greater chance of financial struggle since the person with dementia, and the care partner may eventually have to give up work.
- » May have significant financial commitments, such as school fees, and large mortgages (having planned to work for much longer), and have less financial capital saved.
- » Dependent children may still be living at home, the person may have very young children.
- » Childcare may be required because of the person with dementia not being able to care for their own children, and their partner is still having to work.
- » May have parents who are still alive and who need care.
- » Greater impact of not being able to drive any longer because of work and family responsibilities. For example, not being able to pick up your own children from school or take them or yourself to medical or other appointments; not able to take elderly parents to appointments or on outings.

Greater impact of disease symptoms

- » More aware of their disease in the early stages.
- » Find it hard to accept and cope with losing skills at such a young age.
- » Greater loss of social status, as dementia is seen as an older person's disease.
- » Significant fear of a loss of identity, privacy, and issues such as not knowing your children or grandchildren.

» Reduced self-worth as valued roles are diminished or negated.
» Increased risk of depression, low self-esteem and anxiety.
» Often have the rarer types of dementia (such as frontotemporal or Lewy body) which are less well understood.
» Physically fit and may behave in ways that others could find challenging.

Much less access to services
» There are very few or no age-appropriate services.
» Lack of support for meaningful engagement and pre-diagnosis activities — interests are likely to differ from those of older people
» Services for people with YOD were funded by state governments and now are transitioning to the national disability insurance scheme (NDIS) in Australia. There is currently lack of clarity about eligibility criteria so there is some fear about services being less accessible.

Children of people with YOD

What is it like for young children, when their younger or middle-aged parent is diagnosed with younger onset dementia?

This is one story:

As an only child of a single parent, X recalls seeing changes in his mum from about 8 years old. He lived in a small community where someone labelled his mum, at 42 years old, as a drug addict when they noticed some changes in her. Subsequently, X was no longer able to have friends over to his house. He did not know what was happening to his mum, which he found hard, as he could not explain to others what it was.

He was very protective of his mum and recalls how his friend pointed out to him when he was 11 that he was doing things that a parent normally did. Unknown to him he had started gradually to do things that his mum used to do. It was many years later before he knew her diagnosis of dementia.

When X was about 13 he hung with the 'wrong crowd' and did not attend school regularly. He was sleeping rough at nights to get away from home and drinking alcohol. He knew this was wrong but he needed to escape from his unpredictable home life. There were no boundaries placed on him so he was free to do whatever he wanted. His family and mum's friends no longer visited so basically they were left alone.

They moved to a different area where X was soon labelled a 'trouble-maker' by the first school he attended. He then transferred to another school and it was there that finally a teacher took an interest in him. But the fear of being separated from his mum made him stop disclosing what was happening at home. He recalls having some challenging times at school and felt he did not have much in common with his peers.

Thanks to a supportive teacher he remained at school until year 12 and this provided him with some 'stability' in his life. He did want to go to university but knew this was not going to happen and felt a real sadness about this. A supportive teacher helped him through this time and gave him hope for the future.

They faced financial hardship as there was no money for food and bills so he had to juggle school, paid work and caring for his mother. This eventually took its toll after leaving school where he 'reached a crisis point', he needed to escape and be like his friends — free to leave home.

On reflection he felt he may have been depressed but his focus was on looking after his mum and he felt there was no help for him except to escape to the pub more frequently. He recalls the time when he finally asked for some help, a family member told him that it costs money and he wouldn't be able to afford it, so he did not look into it further at this time.

His crisis worsened and he moved interstate as he wasn't coping, but he organised his extended family to look after his mum before he left. He noted that very soon after leaving, community services were organised to support his mum. He felt lots of guilt but contacted and visited his mother frequently until he eventually returned home feeling stronger in himself to take over her care again. He felt no-one could care for his mum as well as him because he loved her.

This complex and challenging situation continued whilst juggling paid work and his demanding caring role. Finally, with the added benefit of maturity he realised that services and care for his mum was something they were entitled to and not just someone doing them a favour. With this new insight he felt more confident and empowered to get the help they needed. He now recognised himself as a carer and obtained financial support and gained legal advice with regards to managing his mum's financial affairs. He recognised too that he needed a plan for the future. After many frustrating months navigating the complex process of arranging a suitable nursing home placement for his mother, he was successful. He reflected that 'you shouldn't have to jump through hoops to get it' (services and residential care).

When his mum finally was accepted into a nursing home he remembers this time as a particularly emotional and difficult period where he felt he had failed her. He thought his life was spinning out of control but he knew it was time to be her son again. He was able to spend quality time with his mum without all the responsibilities and also finally start to sort out his own life.

'I think having someone to talk to who knew about what was going on, would have made things better for me too. Because I just felt really alone. Didn't feel like I could talk to anyone about that stuff', he reflected.

Chapter 10

We have been told many other stories about young people in a similar situation to the young man above.

Karen Hutchinson has been researching the impact of dementia on young adults and children. Her work identified four common experiences of young people living with a parent with younger onset dementia, which included the emotional toll of caring, keeping the family together, grief and loss and psychological distress. Karen says that children of a parent living with younger onset dementia are often the invisible care partners and are not recognised by health care providers.

Young people have described the impact of having a parent with dementia. They talk of a total disengagement from the world they had known to one of invisibility and fear. 'Escape' from the situation was often seen by young people as the only choice. As a result of the diagnosis, they have experienced mental illness, engaged in drug and alcohol abuse, and even ended up homeless. Many of the young people reported feeling alone, thinking no-one else had a family similar to them. They also had no idea where to get help. One younger person said:

> *There was a big change in the way people treated me when they found out my mother had dementia. Nobody was giving me guidance or monitoring my behaviour. Support from extended family disappears and friends disappear due to the stigma associated with dementia. People don't know how to deal with someone with dementia and distance themselves.*

It is estimated that about a third of patients diagnosed with YOD in Australia have a family member aged under 18 years, however there is no good data on this. There are almost no services for young children of people with dementia.

As the person diagnosed and their care partner are dealing with so many issues, they may accidentally overlook actively supporting their own children. Families sometimes don't speak up about feelings, for fear of upsetting each other, which is normal, but not necessarily helpful for the children of people with young onset dementia And many children won't speak up or ask for help, as they don't wish to upset the parent with dementia.

The overwhelming response of the parents with YOD after attending a workshop run by Karen Hutchinson in Sydney in 2014, is represented by one mother in tears, who said, 'OMG, if I had thought there were few services for people like me, I should have tried being a kid! There seems almost nothing for them, and, it seems, I didn't support them enough'.

She then went on to talk about the feelings of guilt she experienced after the day, and wondered if perhaps, in the rollercoaster of emotions and experiences she herself had felt, she had ignored her own children's needs.

One young adult said; 'I wish I had been given more information, been allowed to come along to the doctors' appointments, so I could ask my own questions.'

One other younger lad said:

> *When Dad had brain surgery everyone at school helped me and my sister heaps, but when he then got dementia, it was like he didn't exist anymore, and no-one bothered with us. I felt like running away and crying all the time, and like they...sort of...thought Mum must be crazy.*

This family needed as much support for a parent with dementia, as for a parent going through any other very serious illness or surgery, and the children talked about feeling stigmatised and isolated by having a parent with dementia.

If you are family member or friend of someone with younger onset dementia, or if you're someone working with dementia within an organisation and you are in a position to support and help the children, it is important you support them proactively. A psychologist, social worker or a case worker would also be helpful but, if that is not possible, then try to find available support organisations for help (e.g. contact Carers in your State/Territory on 1800 242 636 or call Commonwealth Respite and Carelink Centres on 1800 052 222).

Lesbian, Gay, Bisexual, Transgender and Intersex (LGBTI)

People from the LGBTI community will experience some unique encounters or challenges not faced by most others with dementia. Over their lifetime, many LGBTI people report they have accessed routine health care less often than other people out of a fear of being identified as LGBTI, they report they receive inadequate treatment and many say they have faced, and still do face, discrimination.

Many LGBTI couples do not have children, and this can mean there are fewer supports when someone is diagnosed with dementia or caring for a partner with dementia. There is no-one to take the load occasionally, to give you a break. It also might mean that if the care partner gets sick and needs to be hospitalised, there is no support, so being prepared for respite 'just in case', is really important.

Important things to get done early are Power of Attorney, Guardianship and Advance Care Directives. Some health care or service providers may not recognise a gay or lesbian partner as a next of kin, which will make it very difficult when making decisions about health and housing once the person with dementia no longer has capacity.

Consider early on whether you will disclose to a health professional or service or care provider that the person is LGBTI, because as dementia progresses in the person diagnosed, it may affect their ability to conceal their gender identity, sexual orientation or intersex status. Seek out service providers who are sensitive to your needs, and who are publicly making an effort to train staff on sexuality and dementia, as this training usually includes the needs of all sexual preferences, and the staff employed are likely to be less judgemental.

In community care, some have reported having a person who is sensitive to their sexuality and needs makes accepting the service much easier. Residential care providers also need to provide staff who are non-judgemental and who will respect your needs and sexual preferences. If in residential care, and the person with dementia or the couple have not 'come out', it is likely the other residents will notice your sexual preference is different to theirs; humans, even old ones, or those with dementia, still can see and hear, and get a sense about someone they see often.

You may specifically look for residential aged care providers who have been Rainbow Tick accredited. Rainbow Tick accreditation is provided by Gay and Lesbian Health Victoria (GLHV) and the not-for-profit accreditation service, Quality Innovation Performance (QIP). Organisations that are Rainbow Tick accredited are demonstrating their commitment to LGBTI pride, diversity and inclusion. They are letting their LGBTI consumers, staff and community know that they will receive inclusive services from the moment they step through the door. https://www.qip.com.au/standards/rainbow-tick-standards/

If the person's dementia progresses so that they are 'living in the past', the discrimination they experienced when younger may affect how they act about their sexuality. They may become secretive, ashamed, or worried about their sexual preferences, in a way that they were not prior to developing dementia.

There has been very little research on the experiences and needs of lesbian, gay, bisexual, trans and intersex Australians living with dementia. This is partly due to the invisibility of older LGBTI Australians, most of whom grew up in a time when the only way they could protect themselves from discrimination and judgement was to make themselves invisible. The little research that has been conducted suggests that there is a myth that LGBTI people become 'straight' when they develop dementia. There is stigma towards LGBTI people from some aged care staff and the aged care system reinforces traditional social norms about sexuality and is not welcoming of LGBTI people. Based on this research, education resources have been developed to assist providers to create LGBT-inclusive dementia services and are freely available from the Val's Café website at: http://www.valscafe.org.au/

The four-page resource 'We Are Still Gay', is an evidence-based guide to understanding and meeting the needs of lesbian, gay, bisexual and trans Australians living with dementia.

Dementia in people with developmental disabilities

There have been significant improvements in health and social care for everyone, including people with developmental disabilities, which means many are living longer lives. Living longer means that people with intellectual disabilities are more likely to get age-related diseases and conditions, including dementia.

People with intellectual disabilities have unique challenges and needs which increase significantly after a diagnosis of dementia. The other impact is on their parents and families, who have deep concerns about who will support their adult child with a disability after their own deaths, and to add in a diagnosis of dementia makes it more worrying. We recommend you read the book, *Intellectual Disability and Dementia*[33] for information and support if you are in this situation.

Indigenous Australians

Whilst the prevalence of dementia amongst Australia's Indigenous people is unclear, there is some evidence that dementia rates are five times that of the general Australian population.

To date, no studies have examined dementia knowledge levels in Indigenous communities. Dementia is particularly misunderstood in the Aboriginal population, making it less likely they will seek a diagnosis if worried about things such as memory or thinking.

One barrier to dementia care has been the lack of a culturally appropriate assessment tools, which has hindered the evaluation of cognitive impairment in the Indigenous community. The Kimberley Indigenous Cognitive Assessment tool (KICA) was developed and validated in a number of Indigenous communities in the Kimberley region of Western Australia by Dr Kate Smith and Professor Leon Flicker. Alzheimer's Victoria has also done work in this area, and developed tools and resources more culturally appropriate for this group, including partnering with the Winda-Mara Aboriginal Corporation and Indigenous Hip Hop Projects to develop an educational music dance video about dementia for young people. Visit the Alzheimer's Australia website for more detailed information, and their resources.

Many of the first signs of dementia in an Aboriginal person are getting

---

33 *K Watchman*, Intellectual Disability and Dementia: Research into Practice, *Jessica Kingsley Publishers, UK, 2014*

lost on Country, losing stories, forgetting family members, growling, and trouble with cooking and eating. The other important thing to note is that due to poorer health outcomes and reduced life expectancy rates, Aboriginal Australians will be more likely to receive a diagnosis of dementia at a much younger age. Diagnosis and impact can be more difficult for a number of reasons, such as not liking doctors, remote locations and homelessness amongst this group, and fear of what is wrong.

Homelessness and dementia

Rates of homelessness are rising rapidly. There are more than 105,000 people in Australia who are homeless, and the rate of homelessness is 49 out of every 10,000 people, of which 56% are males and 44% female. Older people are at greater risk of homelessness than ever before because of the housing crisis in major cities, socioeconomic disadvantages causing people to be unable to pay bills, rent or keep up with mortgage payments, houses that are 'unfit' to live in and relationship breakdowns. The current homelessness support system does not cater for the needs of older people 'at risk' of homelessness, meaning there are no preventive strategies.

People who are homeless are more likely to develop dementia. In a project currently being undertaken by Clare Beard from Alzheimer's Australia South Australia, she states the dementia risk factors in the homeless are:

- social isolation and lack of mental stimulation
- co-morbidities and dual diagnosis
- head injury
- nutritional vulnerability
- sustained drug and alcohol abuse
- depression
- lack of physical activity
- premature ageing.

If a homeless person develops dementia, this usually leads to a crisis. The homeless person with dementia may have long periods of being unwell, and go undiagnosed, and untreated. There is a lack of awareness of dementia amongst the homeless. Dementia is poorly recognised or understood, brain health is not in the forefront of services as more immediate needs take precedence such as food and treatment for other health issues. Other issues include a lack of an appropriate screening tool, lack of clear pathways for dementia services and access to services, fewer supports, no regular doctor, not being able to afford medication, not taking prescribed medication, not having a fixed address, and the more obvious ones such as time, money and resources.

The other factor facing homeless people with dementia is the stigma of homelessness, which is then coupled with the stigma of dementia.

Beard says we must campaign for awareness, recognise the unique issues they are facing, advocate for equity, work better with agencies and provide services, develop resources for them, and encourage brain-health strategies and risk-reduction strategies.

At the ADI conference in Taipei in 2013, one presenter told the story of a homeless man living in Sydney, who eventually was admitted into residential care as his dementia had advanced to the state of him actually getting diagnosed and assessed for care, which often does not happen for this group. He soon demonstrated 'challenging behaviour', and was bounced from facility to facility as no-one felt equipped to support him.

Eventually someone (from a residential provider) saw this man and agreed to trial providing him with home-care packages on the streets. Whilst this was seen as risky by others, this homeless man had not lived inside a home where the front door was always locked, nor in a single small room, nor been in shared institutionalised accommodation in his whole life, and his aggressive behaviours were simply a reaction to having his freedom taken away. Once he was back living on the streets, with services coming to him, including supporting him with medication, his experience of living with dementia improved considerably and he was no longer violent towards anyone trying to help him. It is a very positive example of consumer directed care being provided to an individual living in way that he chose. Although it may seem irrational to choose to live on the streets rather than in residential facility, to this man being in a facility was worse than being in jail.

People from culturally and linguistically diverse (CALD) backgrounds

Twenty per cent of Australians aged 65 years and over were born overseas in a non-English speaking country. It is estimated that by 2021, 30% of all older Australians will be from non-English speaking backgrounds. People from non-English speaking backgrounds, or born in other countries, or coming from different cultures are collectively referred to as coming from culturally and linguistically diverse (CALD) backgrounds. People from CALD are not a homogenous group; they speak a diversity of languages (and dialects of those languages), and come from many different countries (and there can be differences between groups coming from the same country, for example, people from the Israeli/Palestinian region can be Muslims, Jews or Christians.

Since dementia is associated with decreased cognitive functioning, when a person whose first language is not English develops dementia, the impact of the dementia can be more challenging than for other people with dementia. When individuals from these communities develop dementia, their ability to communicate their needs becomes even more compromised than for someone who is able to communicate through the English language. Often English language abilities are lost before native language abilities.

The top 10 languages other than English spoken at home by people aged 65 and over (in descending order) are:

1. Italian

2. Greek

3. Chinese

4. German

5. Arabic

6. Croatian

7. Spanish

8. Dutch

9. Maltese

10. Polish

Due to the lack of research in this area, we don't know if people from CALD backgrounds get dementia at the same rate (about 6% of the population over 65 have dementia) as Australian born people. This is likely, however, differences in levels of risk factors (e.g. people from Chinese backgrounds have higher rates of diabetes, people from Mediterranean backgrounds are more likely to adhere to the Mediterranean diet) may mean that there are small differences in the prevalence rates in different CALD groups.

People with dementia from CALD backgrounds often present later for diagnosis. This may be because of poorer recognition of the symptoms of dementia, cultural stigma about the disease, belief that it is a normal part of ageing or that nothing can be done.

When a person with dementia who doesn't speak English well presents for assessment, diagnosis can be more difficult. Most cognitive tests are biased against people from non-Western or mainstream backgrounds because of language and assumed knowledge. So people from CALD backgrounds are more likely to do more poorly on these tests and be misdiagnosed with dementia when they don't have dementia. There is a cognitive screening test called the Rowland Dementia Universal Access Screening tool (RUDAS) which is a culturally appropriate cognitive screening tool for use in Australia.

Conducting neuropsychological testing and other cognitive testing using an interpreter is not ideal. The interpreters may not understand dementia or cognitive testing (for instance rather than interpreting the person's exact response to a question, they 'improve' the response, or they give an instruction multiple times when it is only supposed to be given once). Assessors may also not know how to use interpreters effectively.

The presentation of dementia in CALD does not appear to generally differ compared to people without dementia. However, since many people from CALD backgrounds learn English as a second language and speak their native language at home, they 'lose' their English language abilities. This adds to the challenges of communication with medical professionals and aged care staff. Try to find a doctor who speaks the same language or from the same cultural background (or both). In some families even the children and grandchildren may not speak the person's native language well or at all.

People from CALD backgrounds may have experienced trauma in the past, which resurfaces as the dementia progresses. For example, many migrants may have had experiences in the war which impact on how they perceive the world when they have dementia — they may be suspicious of people of other races, be paranoid and hoard food. Someone who was a prisoner of war, may react with anger or fear if 'locked up' in a nursing home. Many older Jewish people with dementia are terrified of having showers because they are associated with genocide during the Holocaust. If you are the care partner of a person with dementia who is a migrant, try and interpret the person's behaviour based on knowledge of conditions during their formative years in their country of birth. Share this information with medical and care professionals.

Our cultural background influences us all. This background impacts on all aspects of our life — how we judge our own way of life and that of other cultural groups, our family structures, beliefs about religion and spirituality, social interactions, how we dress, how we express ourselves, the gender roles of men and women and so on. Another important aspect of cross-cultural communication is the role of the family, as each culture has certain expectations about the roles and responsibilities of different family members. This may include one or more members taking on caring responsibilities for the person with dementia. The ways in which decisions are made within families can also vary considerably across different cultures.

Aged care services for people from CALD backgrounds

People from CALD backgrounds may find it harder to access and use services because of language and cultural understandings. Firstly, they may not know what services are available in Australia, particularly because the health, social and support services provided in their country of origin are so sparse. Sometimes information about services is not available in languages other than English. Even when it is available, the terms used may not make sense, for instance, an older CALD person may not see themselves as a 'carer' or understand what 'respite' is.

People from CALD backgrounds appear to use home care services at similar or higher rates compared to the rest of the population. Consumer directed care allows you to ask for a care worker who speaks your language and comes from a similar background. Currently any translating and interpreting services that you require as part of home care come out of your individual budget, which means that CALD consumers are penalised if they obtain their service from a provider that doesn't have a case manager who speaks their language.

Ethno-specific care

There are aged care services which cater for specific language or cultural groups. This is sometimes referred to as ethno-specific care. Unfortunately, at the time of writing www.myagedcare.gov.au does not allow searching by language or culture, or provide easy-to-find information on organisations that cater specifically for CALD groups by geographical location. One way of accessing information about ethnic-specific services in your area is to contact your state Federation of Ethnic Communities Council of Australia (www.fecca.org.au) affiliates or Partners in Culturally Appropriate Care (PICAC) service. PICAC's are government-funded services which help aged care organisations deliver culturally appropriate care.

- » **New South Wales and Australian Capital Territory**
- » Partners in Culturally Appropriate Care NSW & ACT: www.picacnsw.org.au
- » **Northern Territory**
- » Council on the Ageing Inc (COTA): www.cotant.org.au
- » **Queensland**

- » Diversicare: www.diversicare.com.au
- » **South Australia**
- » Multicultural Aged Care: www.mac.org.au
- » **Tasmania**
- » Migrant Resource Centre (Southern Tasmania) Inc: www. mrchobart.org.au
- » **Victoria**
- » Centre for Cultural Diversity in Ageing: www. culturaldiversity.com.au
- » **Western Australia**
- » Independent Living Centre of WA: www.ilc.com.au

People from CALD backgrounds are less likely to use residential aged care than Australian-born people. There are not enough ethno-specific aged care places, and these are usually only available in urban areas. Life can be confusing and uncomfortable for a person with dementia generally, however, a person from a CALD background with limited-to-no English, living in a mainstream (i.e. not ethno-specific) facility, can be overwhelmed by their environment. Imagine if you were locked in a place where everyone spoke a different language, where the furnishings and food were foreign. You can't communicate, and you don't understand the social norms that everyone else seems to be using. Other residents may get angry at you and yell at you to 'Speak English!'. You don't have anyone to talk to, and can't join in the activities. Nobody understands you, or your needs.

If you're the care partner of someone with dementia from a CALD background, try to get access to ethno-specific services if you can. If you can't, try to find a service where one or more staff members speak their language or share their culture or where staff actually make an effort to support the individual and their family with their specific needs. One of the ways you can assist a person with dementia from a CALD background is to use Communication cards for aged care, (available here in 25 languages www.culturaldiversity.com.au/resources/multilingual-resources/communication-cards) so that staff can communicate more easily with the person.

If in residential care, make up signs in the person's language, remembering that some people are not literate in their own language (www.culturaldiversity.com.au/resources/multilingual-resources/aged-care-signage).

There is a myth that people from CALD backgrounds 'always look after their own'. While traditionally many non-Western cultures place a strong emphasis on family bonds, sometimes these traditions are not as strong post-migration as people assimilate. Families may experience 'culture clashes' between older and younger generations about expectations of care of the older generation, and families may also be spread out geographically.

Chapter 11

FOCUS ON WELLBEING AND QUALITY OF LIFE

A lot of what we've written so far has been about the difficulties, disAbilities and challenges around dementia, but also about positive strategies and practical supports. The public discourse is more often about suffering, and in this chapter we look at the importance of focusing on wellbeing and quality of life instead of only suffering.

We decided to dedicate a whole chapter to wellbeing and quality of life, because living well is about trying to accentuate the positive, not just rehabilitate, support and minimise the negative. We have also included human rights, disability rights and dementia friendly communities in this chapter, as all of these impact on the ability for people to be supported in their communities to live more independent lives, which impact on their wellbeing.

Focus on your quality of life

Positive psychology is a field interested in increasing people's happiness and satisfaction so that they can live meaningful and fulfilled lives. Positive psychology research suggests that we can do things which give us moments of joy, and which increase our levels of happiness, life satisfaction and quality of life.

In order to focus on quality of life and wellbeing, we need to think about the aspects of that we are dissatisfied with or want to improve. Martin Seligman, one of the pioneers of positive psychology has proposed the PERMA model for quality of life. This may help you in thinking about aspects of your life which you may want to devote energy to.

PERMA stands for:

- Positive emotions
- Engagement
- Relationships
- Meaning
- Achievement.

Positive emotions: feeling good, happy, content, satisfied, joyous, peaceful. Research suggests that people who flourish psychologically experience a ratio of three positive emotions to every one negative emotion. This doesn't mean that they don't experience any negative emotion, or only a few negative emotions (they wouldn't be human if they didn't feel sadness or anger!), just that they experience three times as many positive emotions. So try and increase the number of positive emotions that you experience every day. Do things that make you happy, that help you feel peaceful and that bring you joy or give you satisfaction.

You may want to laugh more and do fun things. It is not a waste of time or money devoting resources to feeling good; allow yourself these pleasures, it's good for you! If you find you are not laughing enough, then try joining a laughter club; they can be hilarious fun, and laughing is really good for you.

Engagement: being completely absorbed in activities or experiencing 'flow'. This means that you are so engrossed in an activity that time is irrelevant, as is stress and worry. It doesn't matter what the activity is — it can be work, or play or an everyday task like sweeping the floor. The activity can also be challenging, like a tricky puzzle. Some people find meditation can help them reach this state, and others use mindfulness training. Any activity in which you are 'in the moment' can give you engagement. Importantly, it is best if it has inherent value to you as an individual, and you enjoy it, rather than doing something others think might sustain or amuse you.

Relationships: being authentically connected to others or having meaningful relationships is important; this means that you have intimate, ongoing relationships with people you can trust and rely on. This may mean someone that you can talk to, or someone that you can spend time with doing things together. Spend time nurturing your relationships with friends and family. People with dementia and their families consistently report friends and family members stop calling after a diagnosis, which therefore impacts their health and happiness.

Meaning: having a purpose in life. For many people having meaning involves the service of others, such as caring for your family, or contributing to the community. You may do this in small ways (e.g. making a small donation to charity) or big ways (becoming a dementia advocate like Kate Swaffer and speaking publically about your experiences with dementia and on behalf of others with dementia).

Many people volunteer, and you may find a program which will support your volunteering, or the person with dementia and their care partner might volunteer together. Some people may also find meaning through their spirituality — praying and being connected to God/s.

Achievement: a sense of accomplishment and success. This contributes to your self-confidence and self-worth. The accomplishments and successes could be big things (I built a boat!) or small things (I made a cake!). Many people like to set goals and work towards them, though you don't need to have explicitly set goals to feel that you've done something. If you're no longer working, hobbies and pastimes can often be a source of accomplishment and success. For instance, expressing yourself through art, music, dance or writing.

Prescribed Disengagement may result in reduction in the areas of meaning and achievement, and maybe also in relationships, which would mean a decrease in quality of life, so it is worthwhile finding ways to engage more, rather than disengaging from your life.

For positive psychology resources, including questionnaires to help you evaluate your quality of life and identify your personal strengths, and exercises shown by research to improve happiness, please go to the website hosted by University of Pennsylvania and Dr Martin Seligman www.authentichappiness.sas.upenn.edu.

Below we detail a variety of things that some people do that they find helps them improve their wellbeing and quality of life. There is research evidence behind some of them, which we've noted. Others anecdotally help some people. These are just ideas, so if they don't sound like your cup of tea, that's okay. Try and find things which will help you feel positive emotions, feel engaged and immersed, that nurture your relationships, give you meaning in life and a sense of achievement.

Therapeutic writing

Studies have shown that expressive narrative writing (i.e. writing about personal experiences and feelings) can reduce the symptoms of mental illnesses such as depression and post-traumatic stress disorder. Sometimes putting thoughts down on paper can help us process what has happened and is happening to us, and help us observe how we feel. Writing things down may stop us from going round and round in circles in our thoughts, and help us see insights or move towards a resolution. As we write we take control of the situation, make sense of our experiences and ourselves and cleanse ourselves of our burdens. When writing for others we can engage and connect, improve our relationships, raise consciousness and promote cultural change.

Writing regularly means you also have to use your brain, in other words, give it a neuroplasticity workout, so writing may be good for your brain. Ironically, the latest writing tools, that is, iPads are often referred to as tablets!

Kate writes: 'As long as I write, I feel I can overcome the emotional distress of the symptoms of dementia. Whether it is autoethnography, narrative therapy, or simply, writing for my life, it doesn't really matter'

Here are some ideas for why writing can be helpful:

- » Write about important things from your past — some people write to pass this autobiographical information or family history on to their children or grandchildren, others write to help themselves work through difficult issues.
- » Write about whatever is on your mind, like keeping a

journal or a diary.
» Write poetry.
» Write a letter to someone to express your feelings towards them. You may or may not send the letter — this could be to a loved one, or someone who you are upset at.

When writing for therapeutic purposes, you don't need to worry about grammar or spelling, or other conventions of prose or poetry. You also don't have to reveal your writing to anyone, as the value is as much, if not more, in the expression as it is in sharing it.

Writing an autobiography or having someone help write a biography when first diagnosed with dementia is also a good idea for your family and friends, and can be used for care staff if you ever need respite or residential care. Most people who are diagnosed with illnesses such as cancer or Motor Neurone Disease are provided with a biography service, and this would be helpful for people with dementia as well. In Victoria, there is a serviced called *Beyond words,* who provide a biography service only available for people who live in a Residential Aged Care facility that is within the Melbourne metropolitan area. It is an excellent example of what could be provided, at the time of diagnosis. You can find them here www.beyondwords.org.au.

Autoethnography

Autoethnography is a form of self-reflection and writing that explores the writer's personal experience and connects this autobiographical story to wider cultural, political, and social meanings and understandings. Autoethnography is a technique usually used in fields such as performance studies and English. It has been defined by a well-known autoethnographer as, 'research, writing, story, and method that connect the autobiographical and personal to the cultural, social, and political.' (Carolyn Ellis, 2004)

Writing about living with dementia, or about supporting a person with dementia ensures a strong element of self-reflection, and helps you gain an understanding of this new world of dementia.

Kate wrote about her own blogging and writing:

It has developed from a simple memory bank and legacy to myself and my family and friends, to a social and political voice for people living with dementia, as I seek to describe and systematically analyse my personal experience in order to understand the cultural experience. I think I am attempting to make my personal experience more meaningful and the cultural experience engaging, in ways that now connect with a wider audience than I had ever intended.

Mind mapping

Mind mapping is a graphic technique that is used to facilitate learning and to generate and organise ideas. Mind mapping combines word, image, number, logic, rhythm, colour and spatial awareness. The technique has been shown in research studies to:

- improve memory for new information
- be an interesting and engaging way to process information
- help the person organise and understand information
- help with concentration while learning.

Mind mapping may be useful as a way of thinking or learning about a topic for people with dementia who may find reading, thinking clearly and even comprehension difficult. Kate Swaffer has certainly found it helpful in helping her to plan, reason more clearly and study. There are many online versions of mind mapping, but it can be as simple as having paper, lots of coloured pens and your own imagination.

Belief

Henry Ford once said; 'Whether you think you can, or you think you can't — you're right.'

Dr Bruce Lipton, a renowned cell biologist, in his book, *The Biology of Belief: Unleashing the Power of Consciousness, Matter & Miracles* (2012), will change how you think about your own thinking, and the power of belief. Striking new scientific discoveries about the biochemical effects of the brain's functioning show that all the cells of your body are affected by your thoughts. Lipton's book describes the precise molecular pathways through which this occurs, using simple language, illustrations and everyday examples, and demonstrates how the new science of epigenetics is revolutionising our understanding of the link between mind and matter, and the profound effects it has on our personal lives and the collective life of our species. It is sound justification for believing in Henry Ford's philosophy.

Do you feel helpless in the face of dementia and that the diagnosis controls your life? Or do you feel (like Kate) that there are many things you can do to manage your dementia?

Research suggests that our health beliefs impact our health outcomes. While this has not been demonstrated specifically for dementia, we assume that it also applies to dementia. Health beliefs influence

» How we care for ourselves generally.
» Health promoting behaviour — whether we see the doctor (remember how some people don't think anything can be done about dementia and don't get diagnosed because of this?), whether we take our medication and follow lifestyle and other advice.
» Our physiological systems such as the immune system.
» Our quality of life.

Transcendental Meditation

Transcendental Meditation is a simple and natural mental technique, which is practised for 20 minutes twice a day, sitting comfortably with your eyes closed. It's easy to learn (anyone can learn TM), easy to practise, and doesn't involve any change in lifestyle or any belief system. The word 'transcend' means to go beyond, and in TM, the mind settles down to a state of awareness, beyond thought. During this process the body gets profound rest, in many ways deeper than sleep, which allows accumulated stress to be released.

TM is the most well researched meditation practice in the world, documented in over 350 published scientific papers, in which TM has been shown to be uniquely effective in enlivening brain function and reducing stress-related illness, right from the start of the practice. It is the only meditation recognised by the American Heart Association and the Australian CSIRO to actually lower blood pressure. Other forms or methods of meditation can be helpful as well, although few have as much research into their particular benefits.

Research has found the benefits of practising TM start from the first day and accumulate over time, and has shown benefits in all areas of life, including:

- clearer thinking, increased intelligence and more creativity
- improved health, energy and happiness
- decreased stress, anxiety and depression
- greater efficiency and better relationships at work and at home
- more inner peace, stability and contentment, contributing to a more peaceful world.

The result is clearer, calmer thinking, more energy and less stress. Not surprisingly, this is very helpful for people with dementia and their care partners (there is research to support the benefits for decreasing depression and stress in care partners).

Self-hypnosis (and hypnosis)

Hypnosis is 'a state that resembles sleep but that is induced by suggestion' and self-hypnosis is 'the act of hypnotising oneself.[34]'

A hypnotic process is usually facilitated by a hypnotist, who can also be a medical doctor or a psychologist trained in hypnosis; the hypnotist uses a process of focus and alternative possibilities to distract a person away from, for example, pain. The technique will help the client into a relaxed state through focused guiding by the hypnotist. This technique can be used by the person himself or herself, and can be useful for things like pain relief, and other behaviours, such as losing weight or stopping smoking.

Hypnosis can be used as a technique to manage pain, allowing the reduction of pain medication that has side effects such as drowsiness and being unable to concentrate. It can be helpful for people with dementia who already have reduced cognitive abilities. It doesn't work for everyone, but it is worth trying, especially for people with dementia who are taking pain medication and want to reduce the side effects of that.

---

34 *Free Dictionary http://www.thefreedictionary.com/self-hypnosis*

Mindfulness

Mindfulness is a state where the person has an in-the-moment awareness of his or her own experience without judgement. Mindfulness is usually obtained through exercises such as mindful meditation, though some practices, such as yoga, tai chi and qigong, also cultivate mindfulness. Mindfulness exercises help you to practise being able to identify, tolerate and reduce difficult, painful and even frightening thoughts, feelings and sensations, and can give you back some sense of mastery over your thoughts and feelings. Rather than having the sense that you are being pushed around by your feelings and thoughts you learn to be able to have some control over them.

Research suggests that mindfulness can:

- reduce rumination and worry
- reduces stress and anxiety
- improve positive mood, and decreases negative moods
- helps people not react as strongly emotionally to things that are upsetting
- improve working memory
- improve attention and ability to focus
- help people be more cognitively flexible
- improves relationship satisfaction
- promotes empathy and compassion
- improves overall wellbeing and quality of life
- have some physical health benefits, for chronic pain.

Mindfulness is as simple as becoming aware of your own 'here and now' experience, internally and in the external world around you. It helps you to be able to more positively deal with any distressing and painful memories of things from your past, or it can also allow you to look at and plan for the future, even when you might have fearful thoughts of what is ahead. In the context of someone diagnosed with dementia, there is often a lot of fear for the future, and mindfulness can be really helpful in managing this type of reaction.

There are mindfulness practitioners in most cities and even some regional ones, as well as websites and books where you can read about it, if this is something you feel would be helpful to your own situation. The internet might be your first place to go, adding into the search engine 'Mindfulness practitioners in your city/town'.

Psychosynthesis is a theoretical model of human nature, of the natural unfolding, growing, of the human being. It is based on observation, witnessing and scholarship of the process of biosynthesis. Dr Roberto Assagioli, founder and a contemporary of Freud and Jung, was trained in psychoanalysis. He challenged the limiting view given by Freud to the lower or darker instincts. He introduced the idea of a natural unfolding internal process, which occurred naturally within the very being of the human. Through Psychosynthesis he indicated that this unfolding was as important as understanding how we grow and develop. Assagioli's model recognises transpersonal experiences and the higher qualities of our humanness. His approach is sometimes described as 'a psychology with a soul'.

Psychosynthesis is a positive, strength-oriented approach. Psychosynthesis looks at the whole person. Through the use of meditation and in particular mindfulness techniques it aims to bring balance to approaches that unfortunately focus on pathology and deficit oriented model — this perspective continues to permeate the field of psychology today.

The art and practice of observation and dis-identification means that individuals can observe their mind and realise, that although it may be impaired they can manage the impairment. Through considered care, action new neural pathways may emerge. There are a few practitioners of this technique in Australia, who you can locate from the resource list.

Social media and blogging

You may be surprised by the benefits of using social media for people with dementia and their families. It gives people with memory loss and other cognitive changes other ways to help them recall information, including photographs of the people they are connecting with, as the person's name is always in sight, and the ability to go back to conversations and events later is helpful.

It allows easily accessible, immediate, online support, including support groups, that are available to anyone with the internet, and you can also be part of private Facebook groups, for example, only for people with dementia, or only for care partners. It is possible to speak to someone else in your situation at almost any time of the day and night; this type of online community is truly global, so on the nights when you cannot sleep (and people with dementia have many of these), there is someone in the world who is awake and wants to chat! In many ways, it is an online memory bank, full of your and your friends' lives and activities.

Kate Swaffer realised after starting her blog in 2011, that it really did become her memory bank. It allowed for more meaningful and deeper conversations with her husband, two sons and close friends and it has evolved into a place where there is meaningful dialogue with a wide range of stakeholders about the critical issues impacting a person living with a diagnosis of dementia and their families. Many people with dementia are now blogging regularly, as well as writing books, and getting online to join them is helpful and a lot of fun.

Resilience

Resilience refers to an individual's capacity to successfully adapt to change and stressful events in healthy and constructive ways. Building resilience is important if we are to strengthen our capacity and our skills in order to reduce emotional and mental health problems, and this is important for those of us with dementia, or those of you caring for someone with dementia. It is a skill worth developing as it will give you the ability to overcome obstacles of your past, help you recover from health, career or relationship setbacks and reach your full potential, and it will help you cope with a difficult 'present'.

We all need to encourage personal responsibility, accept more and question less. Accept yourself and your past. Accept your future. If you have dementia, or someone you love or are supporting has it, working on resilience will be really helpful, or the impact of dementia may end up stealing your joy completely and prevent you from living beyond the disease.

Our advice is to work at banning PLOM disease (poor little old me), or you will probably spend too much time with negative thoughts, and not enough time with positive and constructive ones. Live, love and laugh more and worry less. Live every day as if it is your last, just in case it is!

Laughter yoga

Pioneered in 1995 by Dr Madan Kataria, an Indian physician from Mumbai, laughter yoga is a technique which is a scientifically proven method that provides myriad physiological and emotional benefits for people of all ages and abilities. The technique involves doing simple breathing and laughter exercises in a group; these encourage oxygen flow, blood flow and endorphins. Group members may also feel more socially connected through the eye contact and shared positive emotions.

A small group meets in Adelaide occasionally who are using this technique with success. There will be more sessions, including for people with dementia and family care partners, commencing soon.

One older lady with dementia currently doing laughter yoga with her daughter says, 'It is hilarious fun, and I LOVE it!' and her daughter says, 'Her symptoms are much better for about two days afterwards...she wants to do it three times a week!'

Perhaps we all should be doing it?

Lee-Fay wrote, 'I did this once and it was actually great fun and left the whole group feeling energised!'

Getting involved in research

Until recently, research about people with dementia did not often include them, and from the perspective of people living with a diagnosis of dementia, this seems unreasonable. Unfortunately, some researchers still conduct research where they assume that people with dementia can't give their opinions, and they only obtain the views of families or care staff. As people with dementia have started to speak up publicly globally, it is becoming clear that some of the research into the lived experience of patients is not especially accurate, nor valid. Getting involved in research can play a part in being positive and feeling of wellbeing; you and your care partner may feel that it adds meaning to your lives as you are doing something positive for others and the future.

Research incorporating the individual experiences of people living with dementia is on the rise. Reasons for this include recognition that:

- there is a need to address the power inequalities in the relationship between others and people with dementia

- exclusion from the research process can contribute to the objectification and negative, deleterious stereotyping of people living with dementia
- people with dementia are, in fact, capable of expressing their views, needs and concerns, even those who have more impaired language skills
- understanding the lived experiences of people with dementia is important for evidence-based service delivery
- many people with dementia might want to be involved in research
- that people with dementia might actually benefit from being involved in research as participants.

We know that people with dementia usually don't get involved with research. This is not only because of their cognitive disAbilities. There have customarily been people or groups who have been the 'gatekeepers' who have, with the best of intentions, protected people with dementia from researchers. Dementia Alliance International (DAI), which is comprised of an exclusive membership of people living with a medically confirmed diagnosis of dementia, are now working with researchers, to support their work and allow them an easier, more open pathway to connect with people with dementia for research.

If you're interested in participating in research, keep a look out for studies. These may be promoted on the Alzheimer's Australia (or Alzheimer's Australia state organisations') Facebook page, or newsletters. You may also be invited to participate through your doctor or aged care practitioner. Some research studies may only ask a little of your time (e.g. a one-hour interview), others may involve a lot of your time (e.g. if you participate in a lifestyle intervention study over six months with multiple tests including blood tests and brain scans, and exercises to do at home).

People with dementia, care partners and families of people with dementia (often referred to as consumers) may want to contribute by reviewing and critiquing research projects. The Alzheimer's Australia

Consumer's Dementia Research Network (CDRN)[35], is a group of consumers who work with Alzheimer's Australia, the National Health and Medical Research Council, the Cognitive Decline Partnership Centre and Dementia Collaborative Research Centres. Consumers have different roles in research projects — as project leads, collaborators or advisors. The advantages of being involved at this level is that we can influence what research projects are being funded (i.e. encourage the funding of projects that are priorities for us), help to influence the relevance of research, as well as see what is being funded, and how it is translating into practice.

The Alzheimer's Society UK's 'Delivering on dementia: Our strategy 2012–17' published in 2015, states:

> *Everything we do is guided by the seven things people affected by dementia have said they want to see in their lives.*
>
> *1. I have personal choice and control or influence over decisions about me.*
> *2. I know that services are designed around me and my needs.*
> *3. I have support that helps me live my life.*
> *4. I have the knowledge and know-how to get what I need.*
> *5. I live in an enabling and supportive environment where I feel valued and understood.*
> *6. I have a sense of belonging and of being a valued part of family, community and civic life.*
> *7. I know there is research going on which delivers a better life for me now and hope for the future.*
>
> *These are the foundation of our vision, mission and values, and strategic ambitions for 2012–17. Together, we'll make them a reality for everyone affected by dementia.*

It is clear from our conversations with people with dementia and their

---

35 *http://qualitydementiacare.org.au/consumer-network*

families that they want to be involved in research, not only for their own futures, but for the next generations.

Chris Roberts, a man with younger onset dementia from north Wales, who has been taking part in a trial investigating the genetics of Alzheimer's disease said:

> *After a diagnosis of dementia your whole family also receives the diagnosis. It's a team effort. What we then need is hope, and this is what research gives us. Taking part means I'm doing something constructive and worthwhile. I'm leaving something behind that might help others, if not myself. Any kind of research, small or large, brings with it hope that there may be a future.*

Human rights, disability rights and dementia

It is a human right that everyone, including people with dementia, receive best practice, best care, and full inclusion. Too often, and for too long, best practice, best care, and full inclusion has not been the norm.

The very nature of dementia can mean that those diagnosed often have great difficulty in protecting their rights. Society in general has not seen and is not used to this group having a voice, and people with dementia have been shut away and forgotten in society until quite recently. We believe that the lack of general awareness of dementia, and the lack of thorough dementia education in the health care sector is fundamentally an issue of human rights. As such, stigma, isolation and discrimination against people with dementia is still a feature of our lived experience, as we and our care partners and families often report feeling that we are treated with less respect, less dignity and less compassion than other members of society.

The Universal Declaration of Human Rights

The 1948 United Nations Universal Declaration of Human Rights[36] (UDHR) is a milestone document in the history of human rights. To date, even though people with dementia still retain the same rights as anyone else

---

36 *http://www.un.org/en/universal-declaration-human-rights/*

in society, including human rights and disability rights, there has been little advocacy for these rights. However, the recognition of people with dementia under the United Nations Convention of Persons with Disabilities (CRPD) has not been an easy road, and whilst The CRPD includes dementia, the dementia community has not yet used it to claim its rights. Whilst there is positive progress in this direction, which is being made more quickly now, it is still very slow.

As defined by the Australian Human Rights Commission,[37] human rights:

Recognise the inherent value of each person, regardless of background, where we live, what we look like, what we think or what we believe. They are based on principles of dignity, equality and mutual respect, which are shared across cultures, religions and philosophies. They are about being treated fairly, treating others fairly and having the ability to make genuine choices in our daily lives. Respect for human rights is the cornerstone of strong communities in which everyone can make a contribution and feel included.

Most people speak up about the lack of rights on issues such as the testing of animals such as the orangutans for medical purposes, cattle in overseas slaughter houses, prisoners, asylum seekers, people with mental illness. However until recently we did not speak up about the human rights of the infirmed elderly or people living with dementia. When we look at this declaration, we currently fall short for people who are chronically sick, the aged and people who are diagnosed with a dementia. This is changing slowly.

Alzheimer's Scotland has campaigned for some time now to ensure that all legislation, policy and strategies affecting people living with dementia are underpinned by human rights, and subsequently developed their Charter of Rights for people with dementia, in 2009. A human rights based approach is about making people aware of their rights, whilst increasing the accountability of individuals and institutions who are

---

37 *Australian Human Rights Commission, What are Human Rights?, 2013 available at www.humanrights.gov.au/about/what-are-human-rights*

responsible for respecting, protecting and fulfilling rights.

There are some underlying principles, which are of fundamental importance in applying a human rights based approach in practice. These are known as the PANEL Principles.

> » **Participation:** everyone has the right to participate in decisions which affect them. Participation must be active, free, meaningful and give attention to issues of accessibility, including access to information in a form and a language which can be understood.
> » **Accountability:** requires effective monitoring of human rights standards as well as effective remedies for human rights breaches.
> » **Non-discrimination and equality:** a human rights based approach means that all forms of discrimination in the realisation of rights must be prohibited, prevented and eliminated.
> » **Empowerment:** individuals and communities should understand their rights and should be fully supported to participate in the development of policy and practices which affect their lives.
> » **Legality:** a human rights based approach requires the recognition of rights as legally enforceable entitlements and is linked in to national and international human rights law.

In Australia, at the time of writing this book, we don't currently have standards of care. However the first Australian Clinical Practice Guidelines and Principles of Care for People with Dementia have been developed and are available at www.clinicalguidelines.gov.au/portal. People with dementia and their care partners have a human right to better pre- and post-diagnostic care, and to not be subject to discrimination and stigma, in the same way every other group does. It is excellent to see such positive change here and globally.

The United Nations Convention of Persons with Disabilities (CRPD)

People with dementia have been advocating globally for inclusion and recognition under the United Nations Convention of the Rights of Persons with Disabilities (CRPD) for a few years. This advocacy was brought to the WHO First Ministerial Conference on Dementia in Geneva in 2015.

The World Health Organization's position on non-discrimination[38] is important here, as it is often reported that people with dementia are still being discriminated against, and the literature clearly indicates stigma is still high.

> *The principle of non-discrimination seeks 'to guarantee that human rights are exercised without discrimination of any kind based on race, colour, sex, language, religion, political or other opinion, national or social origin, property, birth or other status such as disability, age, marital and family status, sexual orientation and gender identity, health status, place of residence, economic and social situation'.*

Professor Peter Mittler is the Dementia Alliance International (DAI) Human Rights Advisor. His career has spanned more than 40 years working in disAbility rights. Since his own diagnosis of dementia, and his realisation that the disAbility rights of people with dementia were not being recognised, let alone considered, Peter continues to work tirelessly for these rights.

What follows is an edited version of Peter Mittler's introduction to the UN CRPD Convention, with suggestions on how people with dementia will benefit from accessing their right to the CRPD.

---

38 *World Health Organization, Committee on Economic, Social and Cultural Rights, General Comment No. 20, Non-discrimination in economic, social and cultural rights, 2009*

Dementia rights: from words to actions, by Professor Peter Mittler

The time has come for people living with dementia to work in partnership with the wider disability community in claiming their basic rights, as well as those specific to their needs and impairments.

Many fine words are spoken about the human rights of people living with dementia. But very little has been done to enable us to hold governments to account for a recent OECD[39] report that dementia receives the worst quality of care in the developed world.

The UN Convention on the Rights of Persons with Disabilities (CRPD) can do just that. It is the first Convention to have been written in full and equal partnership with the people it is designed to benefit. Seventeen of the 18 members of the UN CRPD Committee that monitors its implementation are themselves people with a disability. By ratifying the CRPD, 159 governments have made a commitment in international law to implement its General Principles and Articles.

People living with dementia across the world are now asking why they seem to have been excluded from this Convention. The simple answer is that they have every right to use it but that only Alzheimer's Scotland has done so to secure a funded guarantee from the Scottish government for a year's post-diagnostic support. Any Alzheimer's Society could do the same.

A new European Commission Dementia Strategy led by Scotland has begun in 2016[40] and the Pan-American Health Organization has just published its plan for the whole Continent[41]. All these plans mention human rights, but none refer to the CRPD as a means of underpinning polices and monitoring outcomes.

---

39 *Addressing Dementia: The OECD Response, Paris, 2015 http://www.oecd-ilibrary.org/social-issues-migration-health/addressing-dementia_9789264231726-en*
40 *http://ec.europa.eu/health/interest_groups/docs/ev_20150319_co04_en.pdf*
41 *http://www.paho.org/hq/index.php?option=com_docman&task=doc_download&gid=31496&Itemid=270&lang=en*

People with dementia still have a long way to go in claiming their rights, but progress is being made.

Dementia friendly communities

A dementia-friendly community is a place where people living with dementia are supported to live a high quality of life with meaning, purpose and value. It is less about being friendly (we should all be like that), and more about respect, human rights, disability rights, non-discrimination, full inclusion, and the right to full citizenship, as well as autonomy, equality, equity, access and dementia enabling environments that support disAbilities.

Whilst health and other services are important for people with dementia to retain their independence, it is also the small things in life that matter to the person with dementia if they are to retain their identity, quality of life and self-respect. Simple things like access to services with staff who understand dementia and have been trained in communication in places like banks, shops and hairdressers.

People with dementia want to be able to continue the hobbies and activities they have always enjoyed, such as fishing or golf, because the broader community including their golf and fishing buddies have some basic understanding of dementia and want to support their friend with dementia.

The physical environment including signage, noise levels, and lighting are also important, as is using respectful language. Access to all supports and services for groups, like those who live alone or are homeless, is an important part of this work. Being dementia-friendly also means providing us with a more ethical post-diagnostic pathway of support, one that is enabling and includes rehabilitation, not disabling and which leads us only to aged care and death. It also means supporting us to be employed, if that is our choice.

Countries and organisations have been working towards the promoting of Dementia friendly communities now for some time. This is relevant for not only the human rights and disability rights of people with dementia and their families, but for things such as accessibility and respect for people with dementia.

Increasing awareness of dementia is a big task, and doing it in a way that is positive and does not further stigmatise and marginalise is also imperative, as some campaigns continue to exacerbate the myth that no-one can live positively with dementia. Understanding the need for full inclusion, respectful positive, and empowering language, and making communities accessible are some of the keys to the success of these campaigns, as well as being some of the biggest hurdles.

Organisations promoting the Dementia Friends or Dementia Friendly Community messages and campaigns need to start within, so that they are actually walking their own talk. A dementia-friendly community must include people with dementia at every step. We recommend that every community or organisation planning to become dementia-friendly sets up a small advisory group of people with dementia, who inform and guide the other organisations and health care professionals involved in the dementia-friendly work.

There are a number of dementia friendly community initiatives in Australia. However the Kiama Dementia Friendly Communities (DFC) Pilot Project is perhaps the best example of authentic inclusion of people not just in Australia but in the world. Established as a partnership between researchers at the University of Wollongong, Alzheimer's Australia and Kiama Council, this project has its own Southern Dementia Advisory Group (who lovingly call themselves the DAG's) of people with dementia supported by their family, friends or a care partner. The project partners, together with people living with dementia and their supporters and interested members of the Kiama community, developed the Kiama Dementia Action Plan in 2015. This Kiama DFC Action Plan is currently being implemented with the direct involvement of the DAG members and other project partners, and the project team just won an Australian National Local Government Innovation award in the Access and Inclusion category.

In closing

There are going to be hard days ahead, whether you are a person newly diagnosed with dementia, or their family or care partner. The dementia will tax you all individually and your relationships.

When you are both especially frustrated with each other and your roles, take some time out, then try and see the situation from the other person's viewpoint. Appreciate how 'hard' it is for the other person. You are both doing your best in a difficult situation, and if you try and give each other a bit of empathy and respect, you may find it less stressful or taxing.

There will be a time when this will be all be up to the care partner and family members, so we recommend you work on things like gratitude and appreciation for each other now, before your loved one's dementia progresses.

If you are the care partner, try to put yourself in the person with dementia's shoes. How would you feel about:

- the idea that you are losing your ability to recall or remember your own life, your children, your friends, the things you did five minutes ago?
- being so confused you can't navigate your way anymore, some days, not even inside your own home?
- not being able to read?
- not being able to spell or write properly?
- not being able to recall the names of artists, paintings, musicians, songs or places you've been before?
- not being able to speak properly, or at all?
- not being able to do simple mathematics or use a calculator?
- living in an aged care facility, a home where you have no key to the front door, and a home where your rights are conditional and you have to become institutionalised?
- not knowing what to do in the toilet, or on the bus, or at the dinner table?
- not knowing who it is on the end of the phone when you pick it up?
- losing your driver's licence and having to rely on others for transport?
- not being able to go shopping alone, let alone get yourself there independently?
- others assuming you are no longer competent at anything?
- being considered as 100 per cent wrong, all the time?

- being confused about how to make a cup of tea, or in what order to shower or get dressed?
- people constantly challenging your diagnosis with comments like, 'But you don't look sick', or 'Your doctors must be wrong', or 'You can't possibly have dementia if you can still function'?
- fighting hard to stay as well as possible for as long as possible, and someone saying you're wasting your time, dementia will get you in the end!?
- being referred to as a symptom, e.g. a wandering or aggressive, rather than the person you still are — Jill, Paul, mother, daughter, friend, nurse, wife or husband?
- not remembering the names of your family or friends, perhaps not even recognising yourself in the mirror?
- If your friends stopped visiting or calling you?
- Being diagnosed with a terminal illness with NO cure, not even on the horizon?

Your care partner may seem to be being overbearing, bossy, and taking away your independence. If you are the person diagnosed with dementia, try and put yourself in your care partner's shoes. Here are some things that care partners and other family and friends have told us:

- I feel so helpless, I don't know how to support them; they won't talk to me about it
- it is awful watching their abilities go
- I find some days it is frustrating being asked the same question over and over and over, after all, I'm human too
- how can I help if they just get angry?
- I just want to hold them tight as I am terrified of the day they won't remember me
- it's so lonely as we used to be so close, and now I feel like a friend and not a husband
- I wish my mum was still acting like my mum and could do all the things other mums do for my friends (13-year-old)
- I am panicked every time they go out alone, even with a

GPS in their phone
- some days I just want to cry all day as I can't bear to think about what is ahead
- moving them into the nursing home was the worst day of my life and I'll feel guilty about it forever; I know I promised I'd never do that, but I was just not able to do it at home any more
- they keep saying their friends never visit; mine don't either
- how do I tell them how bad I am feeling when I know they are the ones who in reality are sick, and can't change what's happening; that would be unfair...right?
- I miss having sex! I really miss it!
- I know the day will come and I'll have to hold their hand when they maybe can no longer swallow, and then I'll have to watch them die
- it will be worse if I'm not there for them when that happens, I don't think I'll ever get over the guilt if that happens
- I hope they remember I love them.

We hope after reading this book you will feel less alone and more able to find support and see what is ahead for you, including how to find services and proactively and positively support yourself. There are millions of people with dementia and care partners out there, and they are facing similar challenges to you. Kate would rather she didn't have dementia, but even though she does, she is living as well as she possibly can, and in spite of the days when she does sit at home and cry.

Most people live for many years after getting a diagnosis of dementia, we hope that you will live beyond the dementia. We especially hope many of the strategies and ideas in this book, and the stories so many people have so generously shared, will support you to live positively for some of the time with dementia too.

It won't be like a special birthday party a lot of the time, and there will be plenty of challenges, but there can be glorious moments of joy along the way.

An introduction to acronyms you might encounter

AA	Alzheimer's Australia
ACAS	Aged Care Assessment Services (Victoria only)
ACAT	Aged Care Assessment Team (Australia except Victoria)
AD	Alzheimer's disease
ADI	Alzheimer's Disease International
BPSD	Behavioural and psychological symptoms of dementia
CALD	Culturally and Linguistically Diverse Communities
CAT Scan	Computerized Axial Tomography scan
CDC	Consumer directed care
CEO	Chief Executive Officer
COTA	Council On The Ageing
CRPD	Convention of Persons with Disabilities
DAI	Dementia Alliance International
DBMAS	Dementia Behaviour Management Advisory Service
DCRC	Dementia Collaborative Research Centre
DTSC	Dementia Training Study Centres
FTD	Frontotemporal dementia
GP	General Practitioner
LBD	Lewy Body dementia
LGBTI	Lesbian, Gay, Bisexual, Transgender and Intersex community
MCI	Mild Cognitive Impairment
MRI	Magnetic Resonance Imaging
Neura	Neura Australia
NHMRC	National Health and Medical Research Council
PET	Positron emission tomography scan
RACF	Residential Aged Care Facility
RDNS	Royal District Nursing Service
SPECT	Single-photon emission computed tomography scan
UNCRPD	United Nations Convention on the Rights of People with Disabilities
VaD	Vascular Dementia
YOD	Younger onset dementia
YOD KWP	Younger onset dementia Key Worker Program

RESOURCES AND REFERENCES

This resource list has been based on resources and websites we felt were the most useful for those who are personally experiencing dementia for the first time. There are, quite literally, millions of websites, including many helpful ones that may not be listed here. Furthermore, new resources, YouTube videos and websites are being created every day.

Organisations

Dementia Alliance International (DAI): the global voice of dementia, and also the peak body globally for people with dementia. DAI is an organisation run by people with dementia for people with dementia. Provides information, educational webinars, online cafes and online support groups.
Go to www.infodai.org for information, www.joindai.org for membership and info@infodai.org for information about their online support groups and others services

Alzheimer's Australia: is the peak body for people with dementia and their care partners in Australia. Provides information (lots of help sheets on their websites), and services including a 24 hour helpline. https://fightdementia.org.au/ National dementia hotline 1800 100 500 (24 hours a day from in Australia)

Palliative Care Australia: http://palliativecare.org.au/

My Aged Care: Federal government website which provides information about government funded aged care services. A searchable database is available. http://www.myagedcare.gov.au/ Call 1800 2000 422 (8am to 8pm Monday to Friday, 10am to 2pm Saturday)

Carers Australia: http://www.carersaustralia.com.au/

Carers Gateway: https://www.carergateway.gov.au Call 1800 0422 737 (8am to 6pm Monday to Friday)

Alzheimer's Scotland: http://www.alzscot.org and **The Scottish Dementia Working Group** http://www.sdwg.org.uk/ the first National Dementia Working Group in the world, started in 2002 and supported by Alzheimer's Scotland. There are now six national Dementia Working Groups, including one in Australia.

Alzheimer's Disease International: the global voice for dementia. Provides information and gives you an idea of international programs, policy and advocacy. http://www.alz.co.uk/

I Can I Will: Alzheimer's Disease International have a library of ideas to help you stand up and speak out about dementia. http://www.alz.co.uk/icaniwill

Useful publications for people with dementia and care partners

Dementia Alliance International, 2016, The human rights of people with dementia: from rhetoric to reality, http://www.dementiaallianceinternational.org/human-rights/

Alzheimer's Australia, 2014, Dementia Language Guidelines, https://fightdementia.org.au/sites/default/files/NATIONAL/documents/language-guidelines-full.pdf

Alzheimer's Australia, 'Talk to me' booklet, produced by people with dementia https://fightdementia.org.au/sites/default/files/TalkToMe_Brochure_FoldedDL_HR.pdf

Dementia Enablement Guide: https://www.health.qld.gov.au/cairns_hinterland/docs/gp-dementia-enablement-guide.pdf

Dementia words matter: guidelines on language about dementia http://

dementiavoices.org.uk/wp-content/uploads/2015/03/DEEP-Guide-Language.pdf

Core principles for involving people with dementia in research

The Scottish Dementia Working Group Research Sub-group (in NHP folder) http://www.sdwg.org.uk/wp-content/uploads/2014/06/Core-Principles.pdf

Risk Guidance for people with dementia

'Nothing Ventured Nothing Gained': risk guidance for people with dementia https://www.gov.uk/government/uploads/system/uploads/attachment_data/file/215960/dh_121493.pdf

The Murray Alzheimer's Research and Education Program (MAREP) has a list of publications, 'By Us For Us' series of guides, specifically for people with dementia, written by people with dementia, found here: https://uwaterloo.ca/murray-alzheimer-research-and-education-program/education-and-knowledge-translation/products-education-tools/by-us-for-us-guides

Useful websites about dementia — with a medical or research focus on types and symptoms

Private Health Care: http://privatehealthcarereports.com/what-is-vascular-dementia-do-you-know-it/

Care Search: http://www.caresearch.com.au/caresearch/tabid/3648/Default.aspx

Videos on YouTube

'Dementia: My Story', What it felt like for Kate Swaffer, not long after diagnosis https://www.youtube.com/watch?v=9ZUyIRq5DAs

Fight Dementia Campaign Rally Speech 2011, Kate Swaffer's first ever rally!

'What is that?' A MUST watch short movie

'If we could see inside other's hearts: Life in 4 mins' A profound look at life in 4 minutes…a 'Must watch'!

Commitment to Care, Adelaide Central Health video

Kids and Dementia: School aged children and grandchildren of people living with dementia have taken part in a series of videos speaking frankly about what it is like having a relative with dementia, in a bid to help other children better deal with the condition. https://www.youtube.com/watch?v=nEJkTMBVMfc&list=PLAwhBH-4GO5iHkEggqw4ruVpkI-Z1GreE&index=1

Son's moving tribute to mum with younger onset dementia: https://www.youtube.com/watch?v=o5QxK0M8OVg

Dementia Alliance International YouTube Channel which has many videos of people living with dementia as well as professional webinars: https://www.youtube.com/channel/UC9OU-TO5MmvYPhmz6j7DYlg/videos

Alzheimer's Disease
Richard Taylor: Alzheimer's from the inside out: https://www.youtube.com/watch?v=EU_aeOqdKIQ and Live outside the Stigma: https://www.youtube.com/watch?v=nyp8rgH4MtU

12 Minutes in the life of someone with AD: https://www.youtube.com/watch?v=LL_Gq7Shc-Y

Apps
Dashlane
SoundNote
Talking Matts

Some other useful resources

Sexuality and Dementia

Alzheimer's Australia (2010), Understanding Dementia Care and Sexuality in Residential Facilities. Freely Available from: https://fightdementia.org.au/sites/default/files/20101001_Nat_QDC_6DemSexuality.pdf

Doreen Wendt-Weir (2006), *Sex in your Seventies*. Learn what the old folk are getting up to; how to cope with a few problems and the expectations of old age. Can be ordered at: www.sexinyourseventies.com

Australian Centre for Evidence Based Aged Care, La Trobe University (2015), 'Supporting families and friends of older people living in residential aged care: A guide for families'. Freely available in Arabic, Greek, Italian, Vietnamese, Mandarin, Spanish, Macedonian and Russian from: http://qualitydementiacare.org.au/project/improving-staff-family-relationships-for-people-with-dementia-living-in-residential-aged-care/ Website also includes education modules for aged care facility staff.

Australian Government, Department of Health and Ageing (2012), National Lesbian, Gay, Bisexual, Transgender and Intersex (LGBTI) Ageing and Aged Care Strategy. Freely available from: https://www.dss.gov.au/sites/default/files/documents/08_2014/national_ageing_and_aged_care_strategy_lgbti_print_version.pdf

Australian Centre for Evidence Based Aged Care, La Trobe University (2014), Sexuality Assessment Tool (SexAT) for residential aged care facilities. Freely available from: http://www.dementiaresearch.org.au/

Hallucinations

Understanding Hallucinations: http://www.alzheimers.net/2014-05-06/hallucinations-and-delusions/

Children's Books

http://www.alzheimers.net/6-03-16-books-for-children-about-alzheimers-and-dementia/ (although most relate to a grandparent with dementia)

Blogs and websites by people with dementia

Kate Swaffer: http://kateswaffer.com/daily-blog/
Wendy Mitchell: https://whichmeamitoday.wordpress.com
John Quinn: https://iamlivingwellwithdementia.wordpress.com
Mick Carmody: http://carmodym59.com
Ken Clasper: http://ken-kenc2.blogspot.com.au
John Sandblom: http://www.earlyonsetatypicalalzheimers.com
Brian Le Blanc: http://abitofbriansbrilliance.com

Blogs and websites by family care partners

Moving your soul, a different way to be with Alzheimer's: http://www.movingyoursoul.com/
Exploring Dementia: http://www.exploringdementia.com
Icare4someone: https://icare4some1.wordpress.com/2015/04/15/64/
The Care-givers Voice: http://thecaregiversvoice.com/about-us/
Dementia Down Under: http://www.dementiadownunder.com

Useful websites for people newly diagnosed with a form of dementia

Lewy Body Dementia (LBD)

Lewy Body dementia association https://www.lbda.org

Fronto Temporal Dementia (FTD)

Australian frontotemporal dementia association — a newly formed organisation http://www.theaftd.org.au/

The association for frontotemporal degeneration http://www.theaftd.org/

Professor John Hodges, Neuroscience Australia (2015) 'Frontotemporal

Dementia: An overview' https://youtube/O0UtwqnHNvo

Managing FTDs and Challenging Behaviours: http://www.blogtalkradio.com/caregiving/2016/07/14/managing-ftds-challenging-behaviors

www.neura.edu.au/FRONTIER
www.neura.edu.au/health/fronto-temporal-dementia
blog.neura.edu.au/podcasts
www.neura.edu.au/research/themes/

Emotional Changes in FTD
https://www.nia.nih.gov/alzheimers/publication/frontotemporal-disorders/introduction
kateswaffer.com/2015/10/09/frontotemporal-dementias
http://www.theaftd.org/life-with-ftd/i-have-ftd/support

Primary Progressive Aphasia (PPA): General
http://aphasia.org.au
http://ftd.med.upenn.edu/about-ftd-related-disorders/what-are-these-conditions/progressive-language
brain.northwestern.edu/dementia/ppa/
http://www.mayoclinic.org/diseases-conditions/primary-progressive-aphasia/home/ovc-20168153
memory.ucsf.edu/education/diseases/ppa
www.ppaconnection.org/index/faq
http://tactustherapy.com/what-is-primary-progressive-aphasia-ppa/

PPA: Semantic
www.theaftd.org/understandingftd/disorders/semantic-dementia
www.aphasia.org/aphasia-resources/primary-progressive-aphasia/
http://www.ncbi.nlm.nih.gov/pmc/articles/PMC2963791/
http://ftd.med.upenn.edu/about-ftd-related-disorders/what-are-these-conditions/progressive-language/semantic-variant-primary-progressive-aphasia-svppa

Putting back the words in Semantic Dementia: https://m.soundcloud.com/neura-podcasts/ep-13-sharon-savage-is-putting-lost-words-back-in-semantic-dementia

PPA: Non Fluent
http://ftd.med.upenn.edu/about-ftd-related-disorders/what-are-these-conditions/progressive-language/progressive-nonfluent-aphasia-pna

PPA: Logopenic

Posterior Cortical Atrophy (PCA)
http://www.brain.northwestern.edu/dementia/otherdementia/pca.html

Other websites:
Frontier: Neuroscience Research Australia http://www.neura.edu.au/frontier

Teepa Snow http://teepasnow.com

Younger Onset Dementia and ME http://youngeronsetdementiaandme.blogspot.com.au

Younger Onset Dementia Association http://www.youngeronset.net/

Alzheimer's Society (UK) http://www.alzheimers.org.uk/

YoungDementia UK http://www.youngdementiauk.org/

Alzheimer Europe http://www.alzheimer-europe.org/

Fisher Center for Alzheimer's Research Foundation http://www.alzinfo.org/

National Alzheimer's Association (USA) http://www.alz.org/index.asp

Alzheimer's Weekly & Dementia Weekly http://alzheimersweekly.com/

The Mayo Clinic Alzheimer's Blog: http://www.mayoclinic.com/health/alzheimers-research-volunteers/MY02005/rss=5

MySimpleC.com: http://href.li/?http://mysimplec.wordpress.com

Dementia and Elderly Care News: Loads of excellent research articles on this site http://href.li/?http://dementianews.wordpress.com

Books
Basting A, *Forget Memory*, The John Hopkins University Press, 2009

Bryden C, *Dancing with dementia*, Jessica Kingsley Publishers, UK, 2005

Doidge N, *The Brain That Changes Itself*, Scribe Publications, 2012

Doidge N, *The Brain Way of Healing*, Penguin Books, London, 2016

Ellison P & Sandlant V (Eds), *The Good The Bad The Brilliant — Lessons from the Journey of Living with Dementia*, Resthaven Incorporated (Free) (2012)

Lipton B, *The Biology of Belief: Unleashing the Power of Consciousness, Matter and Miracles*, Hay House Inc, 2005

Low, LF, add yours in Lee-Fay

Popovic H, *In Search Of My Father*, BookPal, 2011

Power A, *Dementia Beyond Disease: Enhancing Well-Being*, Health Professionals Press Inc, Illinois, 2011

Power A, *Dementia Beyond Drugs: Changing the Culture of Care*, Health Professionals Press Inc, Illinois, 2011

Rahman S, *Living Well with Dementia: The Importance of the Person and the Environment for Wellbeing*, Radcliffe, London, 2014

Rahman S, *Living Better with Dementia: Good Practice and Innovation for the Future*, Jessica Kingsley Publishers, London, 2015

Seligman M, *Flourish: A Visionary New Understanding of Happiness and Well-being*, Free Press, 2011

Swaffer K, *What the Hell Happened to my Brain?: Living Beyond Dementia*, Jessica Kingsley Publishers, London, 2016

Swaffer K, *Love Life Loss A Roller Coaster of Poems*, Kelbane: Graphic Print Group, Richmond, SA, 2012

Tanzi R & Chopra D, *Super Brain: Unleashing the Explosive Power of Your Mind to Maximize Health, Happiness, and Spiritual Well-Being*, Harmony Books, USA, 2012

Taylor R, *Alzheimer's From The Inside Out*, Health Professions Press Inc, Maryland, USA, 2007

Walker R, *The Five Stages of Health*, Transworld Publishers (Division of Random House Australia), 2012

Willis P & Leeson K, *Learning Life from Illness Stories*, Post Pressed, Mt Gravatt, Qld, 2012

Movies

Iris (2001)
The Notebook (2004)
Away from Her (2006)
The Savages (2007)
The Iron Lady (2011)
Still Mine (2012)
Still Alice (2014)

Documentaries

I Remember Better When I Paint (2009)
The Long Goodbye (2010)
Alive Inside: A Story of Music and Memory (2014)
Glen Campbell: I'll Be Me (2014)
Looks Like Laury, Sounds Like Laury (2015)
Alzheimer's: A Love Story (2015)
Still Mine (2012)

Appendix: Summary of Different Dementias

Alzheimer's disease

– Initially, short-term memory loss.
– Getting lost.
– Misplacing things.
– Reasoning, judgement and problem solving, may be more impulsive and less decisive.
– Language, including problems with word-finding.
– Gradual appearance of symptoms.
– Difficulty performing everyday activities.
– Changes in behaviour and personality.
– Depression and anxiety.

Vascular dementias (VaD)

– Great variability in symptoms depending on location of brain damage.
– Changes may be sudden or stepwise.
– When damage occurs deep in the brain:
  • good and bad days, diminished motivation
  • loss of insight
  • poor planning and concentration
  • changes in behaviour and personality
  • poorer judgement

- apathy.
- When damage occurs in the cortex of the brain:
  - memory loss
  - confusion
  - changes in sensory and motor functions
  - language impairment.

Frontotemporal dementias
- Subtypes:
  - behavioural variant — also called frontal variant or Pick's disease
  - semantic variant
  - progressive non-fluent aphasia.
- Behavioural variant (damage more in frontal lobe):
  - personality changes
  - may be disinhibited
  - aggression
  - increased appetite
  - compulsive or repetitive behaviours
  - neglecting usual responsibilities, including personal grooming.
- Semantic variant:
  - loss of understanding of the meaning of words
  - may speak fluently, but describe objects generically e.g. 'thingy'.
  - speech can be fluent but nonsensical.

- PPA variant:
  - loss of ability to find the right words or to speak fluently
  - halting speech, poor grammar, only a few words
  - comprehension may be relatively intact.

Lewy body dementia
- Parkinsonism symptoms such as slowness and decrease in the normal range in movement, difficulty initiating movements, rigidity, resting tremor.
- Fluctuating cognition, especially in alertness and attention.
- Poor problem solving and planning.
- Nightmares or acting out dreams during sleep.
- Visual hallucinations (seeing things that aren't there).

Other dementias
- Dementia associated with Parkinson's disease.
- Dementia associated with Huntington's disease.
- Dementia associated with head trauma (dementia pugilistica).
- Alcohol related dementia.
- Creutzfeldt–Jakob disease.
- Corticobasal degeneration.
- Progressive Supranuclear Palsy (PSP).

First published in 2016 by New Holland Publishers Pty Ltd
London • Sydney • Auckland

The Chandlery Unit 704 50 Westminster Bridge Road London SE1 7QY United Kingdom
1/66 Gibbes Street Chatswood NSW 2067 Australia
5/39 Woodside Ave Northcote, Auckland 0627 New Zealand

www.newhollandpublishers.com

A record of this book is held at the British Library and the National Library of Australia.

ISBN 9781742576442

Managing Director: Fiona Schultz
Publisher: Diane Ward
Project Editor: Liz Hardy
Designer: Andrew Quinlan
Cover Design: Andrew Quinlan
Production Director: James Mills-Hicks
Printer: Hang Tai Printing
10 9 8 7 6 5 4 3 2 1

Keep up with New Holland Publishers on Facebook
www.facebook.com/NewHollandPublishers